PURPLE PLAN COOKBOOK

150+ QUICK & EASY RECIPES FOR BEGINNERS TO QUICKLY BURN
REGAIN YOUR HEALTH | THE ULTIMATE MEAL PLAN FOR A SLIMMER, HEALTHIER YOU

Table of Contents

Introduction

Human health is one of the most important aspects of life. There are many diets that are around to help people recover their health, but few compare to Purple Plan diet.

Purple Plan contains all the nutrients and vitamins an average human needs in a day. Additionally, it is low on calories so that people can still eat without feeling guilty about binge eating or experiencing weight gain.

Purple Plan is a revolutionary diet that offers people the chance to lose weight and stay healthy. It can even help people with other health problems, such as high blood pressure and constant inflammation in the body.

Purple Plan contains all nutrients necessary for a healthy daily life. It has ingredients that stimulate metabolism, maintain blood pressure, prevent cholesterol buildup in the human bloodstream and keep away weight gain.

Another benefit of the Purple Plan diet is that it contains foods from all food groups in an appropriate amount. This way people will receive all the vitamins and minerals necessary to stay healthy even with the reduced quantities from food.

The Purple Plan diet has been tested by many professionals and it has proven to be extremely effective. People on this diet have managed to lose weight in a healthy way without undergoing any type of surgery or any other unhealthy methods for reducing weight.

It is a natural diet that has positive effects on human health. It can regularly be used as a supplement to medicine or as part of an overall healthy lifestyle.

Purple Plan diet is a healthy way to maintain a healthy lifestyle. It is unlike other diets that alter human food habits and food intake. The ingredients used in this diet are all natural and can be found in nature. With the help of these ingredients, people will be able to maintain their weight without experiencing any side effects.

The Purple Plan diet is made up of natural ingredients; therefore it has no negative side effects on health or body weight control.

Studies have been conducted with this diet, and there were no negative side effects. Many people that used the Purple Plan diet manage to lose between 5 and 10 pounds in a month's time. However, people can also lose up to 20 pounds in a month's period if they are dedicated to losing weight.

Purple Plan encourages people to eat healthy without having to eat less than they need. Instead of starving themselves, people can still eat without having to worry about gaining weight.

These days, people are more concerned about losing weight than they are about gaining it. That is why the Purple Plan diet is so popular. It has been proven to be very effective for those that want to lose weight without risking their health or endangering their life.

People that decide to go on a diet often do not know what they can eat and what they shouldn't. Because of this, some individuals resort to unhealthy diets that will only lead to weight gain later on. The Purple Plan diet is unlike any other because it gives people a list of ingredients that they can eat and those that they must avoid. This makes the Purple Plan diet more reliable than other diets.

As people get older, they often gain weight. This leads to many health issues and diseases. The Purple Plan diet will help in preventing high calorie intake which can lead to weight gain in the long term. Therefore, people will be able to maintain their weight without any problems .

The Purple Plan diet has a great impact on the human body as a whole. It can help manage cholesterol levels, blood pressure, and other health problems that can arise with age or improper diet. By maintaining the correct body weight, people will be able to prevent many serious health conditions.

The Purple Plan diet is beneficial not only for weight management but also for helping people with other health issues. It can help control blood sugar levels in diabetics and it is great in preventing strokes and even heart attacks. It's great for those who want to live longer and healthier lives.

Purple Plan is a great choice for people that want to maintain their weight, but it can also be used by people that have other health problems. The food intake from this plan helps manage blood pressure, cholesterol and body weight.

When people use the Purple Plan diet, they can be certain that they will not experience any of the negative side effects of such a drastic diet. The ingredients used in the diet are all natural and have proven to be effective for weight loss.

The Purple Plan diet has been developed by nutritionists and other health professionals after many years of research. It's a great diet that is easy to follow, even by people with busy lifestyles.

Chapter 1.   Breakfast Recipes

1.   Potato Pancakes

Preparation time: 10 minutes

Cooking time: 20 minutes

Servings: 10

Ingredients:

- ½ cup white whole-wheat flour
- 3 large potatoes, grated
- ½ of a medium white onion, peeled, grated
- 1 jalapeno, minced
- 2 green onions, chopped
- 1 tablespoon minced garlic
- 1 teaspoon salt
- ¼ teaspoon baking powder
- ¼ teaspoon ground pepper
- 4 tablespoons olive oil

Directions:

1. Take a large bowl, place all the ingredients except for oil and then stir until well combined; stir in 1 to 2 tablespoons water if needed to mix the batter.
2. Take a large skillet pan, place it over medium-high heat, add 2 tablespoons of oil and then let it heat.
3. Scoop the pancake mixture in portions into the pan, shape each portion like a pancake and then cook for 5 to 7 minutes per side until pancakes turn golden brown and thoroughly cooked.
4. When done, transfer the pancakes to a plate, add more oil into the pan and then cook more pancakes in the same manner. Serve straight away.

Nutrition:

Calories: 69

Fat: 1 g

Protein: 2 g

Carbs: 12 g

2.   Chocolate Chip Pancakes

Preparation time: 5 minutes

Cooking time: 10 minutes

Servings: 6

Ingredients:

- 1 cup white whole-wheat flour
- ½ cup chocolate chips, vegan, unsweetened
- 1 tablespoon baking powder
- ¼ teaspoon salt
- 2 teaspoons coconut sugar
- 1 ½ teaspoon vanilla extract, unsweetened
- 1 cup almond milk, unsweetened
- 2 tablespoons coconut butter, melted
- 2 tablespoons olive oil

Directions:

1. Take a large bowl, place all the ingredients except for oil and chocolate chips, and then stir until well combined. Add chocolate chips, and then fold until just mixed.

2. Take a large skillet pan, place it over medium-high heat, add 1 tablespoon oil and then let it heat.
3. Scoop the pancake mixture in portions into the pan, shape each portion like a pancake and then cook for 5 to 7 minutes per side until pancakes turn golden brown and thoroughly cooked.
4. When done, transfer the pancakes to a plate, add more oil into the pan and then cook more pancakes in the same manner. Serve straight away.

Nutrition:

Calories: 172

Fat: 6 g

Protein: 2.5 g

Carbs: 28 g

3. Turmeric Steel-Cut Oats

Preparation time: 5 minutes

Cooking time: 10 minutes

Servings: 2

Ingredients:

- ½ cup steel-cut oats
- 1/8 teaspoon salt
- 2 tablespoons maple syrup
- ½ teaspoon ground cinnamon
- 1/3 teaspoon turmeric powder
- ¼ teaspoon ground cardamom
- ¼ teaspoon olive oil
- 1 ½ cups water
- 1 cup almond milk, unsweetened

For the Topping:

- 2 tablespoons pumpkin seeds
- 2 tablespoons chia seeds

Directions:

1. Take a medium saucepan, place it over medium heat, add oats, and then cook for 2 minutes until toasted. Pour in the milk plus water, stir until mixed, and then bring the oats to a boil.
2. Then switch heat to medium-low level, simmer the oats for 10 minutes, and add salt, maple syrup, and spices.
3. Stir until combined, cook the oats for 7 minutes or more until cooked to the desired level and when done, let the oats rest for 15 minutes.
4. When done, divide oats evenly between two bowls, top with pumpkin seeds and chia seeds and then serve.

Nutrition:

Calories: 234

Fat: 4 g

Protein: 7 g

Carbs: 41 g

4. Cheesy Jackfruit Chilaquiles

Preparation time: 5 minutes

Cooking time: 20 minutes

Servings: 4

Ingredients:

- 4 (6-inch) corn tortillas, each cut into 8 strips

- 3 tablespoons aquafaba
- 1 (14.5-ounce) can diced tomatoes
- 1 cup Vegetable Broth
- 4 garlic cloves
- 1 teaspoon chili powder
- 1 teaspoon cayenne pepper
- 1 teaspoon ground cumin
- 1 teaspoon dried Mexican oregano
- 1 (14-ounce) can jackfruit, drained
- 1 cup Cheesy Chickpea Sauce

Directions:

1. Preheat the oven to 350°F. Prepare your baking sheet lined using a parchment paper or a silicone baking mat.
2. In a bowl, combine the tortillas and aquafaba and toss until the strips are completely coated. Place the tortillas in a single layer on the prepared baking sheet and bake for 15 minutes.
3. In a blender, combine the tomatoes, broth, chili powder, cayenne pepper, cumin, oregano, and purée. Pour the mixture into a large skillet and bring to a boil over medium-high heat.
4. Add the jackfruit to the sauce and return the sauce to a boil. Lower the heat to medium. Add the tortilla strips, gently stir until coated, cover, and cook until the tortillas are slightly soft but still crunchy, 2 to 3 minutes more.
5. Spoon into four bowls. Drizzle about ½ cup of the chickpea sauce over each bowl, if desired, and serve.

Nutrition:

Calories: 253

Fat: 3g

Protein: 8g

Carbs: 52g

5. Keto Porridge

Preparation time: 15 minutes

Cooking time: 10 minutes

Servings: 1

Ingredients:

- ½ tsp vanilla extract
- ¼ tsp granulated stevia
- 1 tbsp chia seeds
- 1 tbsp flaxseed meal
- 2 tbsp unsweetened shredded coconut
- 2 tbsp almond flour
- 2 tbsp hemp hearts
- ½ cup of water
- Pinch of salt

Directions:

1. Add all fixings except vanilla extract to a saucepan and heat over low heat until thickened. Stir well and serve warm.

Nutrition:

Calories 370

Fat 30.2 g

Carbohydrates 12.8 g

Protein 13.5 g

6. Chia Seed Pudding

Preparation time: 15 minutes

Cooking time: 0 minutes

Servings: 4

Ingredients:

- ¼ tsp. cinnamon
- 15 drops liquid stevia
- ½ tsp. vanilla extract
- ½ cup chia seeds
- 2 cups unsweetened coconut milk

Directions:

1. Add all ingredients into the glass jar and mix well. Close jar with lid and place in the refrigerator for 4 hours. Serve chilled and enjoy.

Nutrition:

Calories 347

Fat 33.2 g

Carbohydrates 9.8 g

Protein 5.9 g

7. Vegan Zoodles

Preparation time: 15 minutes

Cooking time: 10 minutes

Servings: 4

Ingredients:

- 4 small zucchinis, spiralized into noodles
- 3 tbsp vegetable stock
- 1 cup red pepper, diced
- 1/2 cup onion, diced
- 3/4 cup nutritional yeast
- 1 tbsp garlic powder
- Pepper

- Salt

Directions:

1. Add zucchini noodles, red pepper, and onion in a pan with vegetable stock and cook over medium heat for a few minutes.
2. Add nutritional yeast and garlic powder and cook for few minutes until creamy—season with pepper and salt. Stir well and serve.

Nutrition:

Calories 71

Fat 0.9 g

Carbohydrates 12.1 g

Protein 5.7 g

8. Avocado Tofu Scramble

Preparation time: 15 minutes

Cooking time: 7 minutes

Servings: 1

Ingredients:

- 1 tbsp fresh parsley, chopped
- ½ medium avocado
- ½ block firm tofu drained and crumbled
- ½ cup bell pepper, chopped
- ½ cup onion, chopped
- 1 tsp olive oil
- 1 tbsp water
- ¼ tsp cumin
- ¼ tsp garlic powder
- ¼ tsp paprika
- ¼ tsp turmeric

- 1 tbsp nutritional yeast
- Pepper
- Salt

Directions:

1. In a bowl, mix nut yeast, water, and spices. Put it separately. Now heat the olive oil to the pan over medium heat.
2. Add onion and bell pepper and sauté for 5 minutes. Add crumbled tofu and nutritional yeast to the pan and sauté for 2 minutes. Top with parsley and avocado. Serve and enjoy.

Nutrition:

Calories 164

Fat 9.7 g

Carbohydrates 15 g

Protein 7.4 g

9. Tofu Fries

Preparation time: 15 minutes

Cooking time: 20 minutes

Servings: 4

Ingredients:

- 15 oz firm tofu, drained, pressed, and cut into long strips
- ¼ tsp garlic powder
- ¼ tsp onion powder
- ¼ tsp cayenne pepper
- ¼ tsp paprika
- ½ tsp oregano
- ½ tsp basil
- 2 tbsp olive oil

- Pepper
- Salt

Directions:

1. Warm oven to 375 F. Add all ingredients into the large mixing bowl and toss well. Place marinated tofu strips on a baking tray and bake in a preheated oven for 20 minutes.
2. Turn tofu strips to the other side and bake for another 20 minutes. Serve and enjoy.

Nutrition:

Calories 137

Fat 11.5 g

Carbohydrates 2.3 g

Protein 8.8 g

10. Chia Raspberry Pudding Shots

Preparation time: 1 hour & 15 minutes

Cooking time: 0 minutes

Servings: 4

Ingredients:

- ½ cup raspberries
- 10 drops liquid stevia
- 1 tbsp unsweetened cocoa powder
- ¼ cup unsweetened almond milk
- ½ cup unsweetened coconut milk
- ¼ cup chia seeds

Directions:

1. Add all ingredients into the glass jar and stir well to combine. Pour pudding

mixture into the shot glasses and place in the refrigerator for 1 hour. Serve chilled and enjoy.

Nutrition:

Calories 117

Fat 10 g

Carbohydrates 5.9 g

Protein 2.7 g

11. Chia-Almond Pudding

Preparation time: 60 minutes

Cooking time: 0 minutes

Servings: 2

Ingredients:

- ½ tsp vanilla extract
- ¼ tsp almond extract
- 2 tbsp ground almonds
- 1 ½ cups unsweetened almond milk
- ¼ cup chia seeds

Directions:

1. Add chia seeds in almond milk and soak for 1 hour. Add chia seed and almond milk into the blender.
2. Add remaining ingredients to the blender and blend until smooth and creamy. Serve and enjoy.

Nutrition:

Calories 138

Fat 10.2 g

Carbohydrates 6 g

Protein 5.1 g

12. Fresh Berries with Cream

Preparation time: 15 minutes

Cooking time: 0 minutes

Servings: 1

Ingredients:

- 1/2 cup coconut cream
- 1 oz strawberries
- 1 oz raspberries
- 1/4 tsp vanilla extract

Directions:

1. Add all fixings into the blender and blend until smooth. Pour in serving bowl and top with fresh berries. Serve and enjoy.

Nutrition:

Calories 303

Fat 28.9 g

Carbohydrates 12 g

Protein 3.3 g

13. Almond Hemp Heart Porridge

Preparation time: 15 minutes

Cooking time: 5 minutes

Servings: 2

Ingredients:

- ¼ cup almond flour
- ½ tsp cinnamon
- ¾ tsp vanilla extract
- 5 drops stevia

- 1 tbsp chia seeds
- 2 tbsp ground flax seed
- ½ cup hemp hearts
- 1 cup unsweetened coconut milk

Directions:

1. Add all ingredients except almond flour to a saucepan. Stir to combine. Heat over medium heat until it just starts to boil lightly.
2. Once start bubbling, then stir well and cook for 1 minute more. Remove from heat and stir in almond flour. Serve immediately and enjoy.

Nutrition:

Calories 329

Fat 24.4 g

Carbohydrates 9.2 g

Protein 16.2 g

14. Cauliflower Zucchini Fritters

Preparation time: 15 minutes

Cooking time: 10 minutes

Servings: 4

Ingredients:

- 3 cups cauliflower florets
- ¼ tsp black pepper
- ¼ cup coconut flour
- 2 medium zucchinis, grated and squeezed
- 1 tbsp coconut oil
- ½ tsp sea salt

Directions:

1. Steam cauliflower florets for 5 minutes. Add cauliflower into the food processor and process until it looks like rice.
2. Add all ingredients except coconut oil to the large bowl and mix until well combined. Make small round patties from the mixture and set them aside.
3. Heat coconut oil in a pan over medium heat. Place patties on pan and cook for 3-4 minutes on each side. Serve and enjoy.

Nutrition:

Calories 68

Fat 3.8 g

Carbohydrates 7.8 g

Protein 2.8 g

15. Chocolate Strawberry Milkshake

Preparation time: 5 minutes

Cooking time: 0 minutes

Servings: 2

Ingredients:

- 1 cup of ice cubes
- ¼ cup unsweetened cocoa powder
- 2 scoops of vegan protein powder
- 1 cup strawberries
- 2 cups unsweetened coconut milk

Directions:

1. Add all fixings into the blender and blend until smooth and creamy. Serve immediately and enjoy.

Nutrition:

Calories 221

Fat 5.7 g

Carbohydrates 15 g

Protein 27.7 g

16. Ginger Chocolate Oats

Preparation Time: 3 minutes

Cooking time: 0 minutes

Servings: 1

Ingredients:

- 2 tablespoon chocolate chips
- 1 ¾ oz rolled oats
- 1 cup almond milk
- 1 tablespoon cocoa
- 1/2 teaspoon ground ginger
- 1 tablespoon chia seeds
- 1 tablespoon maple syrup

Directions:

1. In a sealable jar or container, place all fixings; put the milk last. Stir the mixture properly and cover. With the jar covered, shake properly to mix the fixings. Keep the jar refrigerated for about 6 hours.

Nutrition:

Calories: 347

Carbs: 56g

Protein: 17g

Fat: 12g

17. Pumpkin Spice Oatmeal

Preparation time: 5 minutes

Cooking time: 8 minutes

Servings: 2

Ingredients:

- ¼ cup Medjool dates, pitted, chopped
- 2/3 cup rolled oats
- 1 tablespoon maple syrup
- ½ teaspoon pumpkin pie spice
- ½ teaspoon vanilla extract, unsweetened
- 1/3 cup pumpkin puree
- 2 tablespoons chopped pecans
- 1 cup almond milk, unsweetened

Directions:

1. Take a medium pot, place it over medium heat, and then add all the ingredients except for pecans and maple syrup.
2. Stir all the ingredients until combined, and then cook for 5 minutes until the oatmeal has absorbed all the liquid and thickened.
3. When done, divide oatmeal evenly between two bowls, top with pecans, drizzle with maple syrup and then serve.

Nutrition:

Calories: 175

Fat: 3.2 g

Protein: 5.8 g

Carbs: 33 g

18. Peanut Butter Bites

Preparation time: 15 minutes

Cooking time: 0 minutes

Servings: 20 balls

Ingredients:

- 1 cup rolled oats
- 12 Medjool dates, pitted
- ½ cup peanut butter, sugar-free

Directions:

1. Plug in a blender or a food processor, add all the ingredients in its jar, and then cover with the lid. Pulse for 5 minutes until well combined, and then tip the mixture into a shallow dish.
2. Shape the mixture into 20 balls, 1 tablespoon of mixture per ball, and then serve.

Nutrition:

Calories: 103.1

Fat: 4.3 g

Protein: 2.3 g

Carbs: 15.4 g

19. Maple and Cinnamon Overnight Oats

Preparation time: 2 hours & 15 minutes

Cooking time: 0 minutes

Servings: 4

Ingredients:

- 2 cups rolled oats
- ¼ cup chopped pecans
- ¾ teaspoon ground cinnamon
- 1 teaspoon vanilla extract, unsweetened
- 3 tablespoons coconut sugar
- 3 tablespoons maple syrup
- 2 cups almond milk, unsweetened

Directions:

1. Take four mason jars, and then add ½ cup oats, ¼ teaspoon vanilla, and ½ cup milk.
2. Take a small bowl, add maple syrup, cinnamon, and sugar, stir until mixed, add this mixture into the oats mixture and then stir until combined.
3. Cover the jars with the lid and then let them rest in the refrigerator for a minimum of 2 hours or more until thickened.
4. When ready to eat, top the oats with pecans, sprinkle with cinnamon, drizzle with maple syrup and then serve.

Nutrition:

Calories: 292

Fat: 9 g

Protein: 7 g

Carbs: 48 g

20. Beans on Toast

Preparation time: 5 minutes

Cooking time: 10 minutes

Servings: 4

Ingredients:

- 2 cups cooked navy beans
- 1/3 cup sun-dried tomatoes, chopped
- ½ of a medium white onion, peeled, chopped
- 1 teaspoon minced garlic
- 1 tablespoon molasses
- 2 teaspoons soy sauce
- ¼ cup tomato paste
- ¼ cup ketchup
- ¼ teaspoon liquid smoke
- 1 tablespoon olive oil
- ¼ cup of water
- 4 slices of whole-wheat bread

Directions:

1. Take a large skillet pan, place it over medium-high heat, add oil and then let it heat. Add onion, stir in garlic and then cook for 5 minutes until onion begins to brown.
2. Add remaining ingredients except for bread slices, stir until combined, and then cook the mixture for 5 minutes or more until thoroughly hot. Spread the bean batter over the bread slices and then serve.

Nutrition:

Calories: 290

Fat: 6 g

Protein: 9 g

Carbs: 51 g

21.   Gluten Free Pancakes

Preparation Time: 10 minutes

Cooking time: 5 minutes

Servings: 6

Ingredients:

- 1 cup almond milk, unsweetened
- 1 filled cup cornflour
- 4 teaspoon vanilla extract
- 1 tablespoon baking powder
- 4 teaspoon sugar
- 1/2 teaspoon salt
- Vegan butter

Directions:

1. In a medium bowl, place baking powder, sugar, cornflour, and salt. Using a whisk, mix these Ingredients: properly.
2. Next, add milk and vanilla to the bowl and continue mixing. Place a skillet over medium-low heat—grease pan with vegan butter. Add the contents of your bowl to the skillet, a third of a cup at a time.
3. Cook each side for about 2 minutes. The sides of the pancakes should be set, and bubbles should be noticeable on top.
4. Use a spatula and be gentle when flipping the pancakes. Take them from the pan, and they're ready to serve.

Nutrition:

Calories: 95

Carbs: 19g

Protein: 1/2g

Fat: 1.3

22.   Carrot Cake Quinoa Flake Protein Loaf

Preparation Time: 9 minutes

Cooking time: 6 minutes

Servings: 2

Ingredients:

- 1/2 cup quinoa flakes
- 1/2 cup grated carrots
- 1 1/2 tablespoon protein powder
- 1 teaspoon orange zest
- Pinch salt
- 1/2 cup almond milk, unsweetened
- 4 packets natural sweetener of choice
- 1/3 cup applesauce, unsweetened
- 1 teaspoon ground cinnamon

Directions:

1. In a mini loaf pan, coat with cooking spray. In a medium-sized bowl, add the natural sweeteners, carrots, cinnamon, zest, applesauce, salt, and almond milk. Stir the fixings well.
2. Add protein powder and quinoa flakes. Stir well to incorporate them into the other fixings before putting the entire batter into the loaf pan. Pat the top to make it even.
3. Cook in the microwave within 6 minutes. Your dessert is ready when the top is firm. Set aside to cool before serving.

Nutrition:

Calories: 165

Carbs: 26g

Protein: 9.5g

Fat: 2.5g

Chapter 2.   Lunch Recipes

23.   Lettuce Wraps with Smoked Tofu

Preparation time: 15 minutes

Cooking time: 25 minutes

Servings: 4

Ingredients:

- 1 (13-ounce) package organic, extra-firm smoked tofu, drained and cubed
- 1 tablespoon coconut oil
- ½ cup yellow onion, finely chopped
- 3 celery stalks, finely chopped
- 1 red bell pepper, chopped
- Pinch salt
- 1 cup cremini mushrooms, finely chopped
- 1 garlic clove, minced
- ½ teaspoon ginger, minced
- 3 tablespoons Bragg Liquid Aminos, coconut aminos, or tamari
- ½ teaspoon red pepper flakes
- Freshly ground black pepper
- 8 to 10 large romaine leaves, washed and patted dry

Directions:

1. Preheat the oven to 350°F. Prepare a baking sheet lined using parchment paper or a silicone liner; then place the tofu cubes in a single layer. Bake the

tofu cubes for 25 minutes, flipping them after 10 to 15 minutes. Set aside.

2. Meanwhile, warm the coconut oil in a nonstick sauté pan over medium-high heat. Add the onion, celery, bell pepper, and salt and cook for about 5 minutes or until the onions are slightly translucent.

3. Add the mushrooms, garlic, and ginger and sauté for about 5 minutes more or until the mushrooms begin to release water. Adjust the heat to medium, then put the aminos or tamari and the red pepper flakes.

4. Add the baked tofu cubes to the pan and sprinkle with pepper. Sauté for a few minutes more, until the tofu is coated with sauce and the veggies are tender.

5. To serve, scoop as much of the veggie and tofu mixture into each romaine leaf as you'd like.

Nutrition:

Calories: 160

Fat: 8g

Carbohydrate: 6g

Protein: 14g

24. Brussels Sprouts & Cranberries Salad

Preparation Time: 10minutes

Cooking Time: 0 minute

Servings: 6

Ingredients:

- 3 tablespoons lemon juice

- ¼ cup olive oil
- Salt and pepper to taste
- 1 lb. Brussels sprouts, sliced thinly
- ¼ cup dried cranberries, chopped
- ½ cup pecans, toasted and chopped
- ½ cup Parmesan cheese shaved

Direction

1. Mix the lemon juice, olive oil, salt, and pepper in a bowl. Toss the Brussels sprouts, cranberries, and pecans in this mixture. Sprinkle the Parmesan cheese on top.

Nutrition:

Calories 245

Fat 18.9 g

Carbohydrate 15.9 g

Protein 6.4 g

25. Quinoa Avocado Salad

Preparation Time: 15 minutes

Cooking Time: 4 minutes

Servings: 4

Ingredients:

- 2 tablespoons balsamic vinegar
- ¼ cup cream
- ¼ cup buttermilk
- 5 tablespoons freshly squeezed lemon juice, divided
- 1 clove garlic, grated
- 2 tablespoons shallot, minced
- Salt and pepper to taste
- 2 tablespoons avocado oil, divided

- 1 ¼ cups quinoa, cooked
- 2 heads endive, sliced
- 2 firm pears, sliced thinly
- 2 avocados, sliced
- ¼ cup fresh dill, chopped

Direction

1. Combine the vinegar, cream, milk, 1 tablespoon lemon juice, garlic, shallot, salt, and pepper in a bowl. Pour 1 tablespoon oil into a pan over medium heat. Heat the quinoa for 4 minutes.
2. Transfer quinoa to a plate. Toss the endive and pears in a mixture of remaining oil, remaining lemon juice, salt, and pepper. Transfer to a plate.
3. Toss the avocado in the reserved dressing. Add to the plate. Top with the dill and quinoa.

Nutrition:

Calories: 431

Fat: 28.5g

Carbohydrates: 42.7g

Protein:6.6g

26. Roasted Sweet Potatoes

Preparation Time: 20 minutes

Cooking Time: 20 minutes

Servings: 4

Ingredients:

- 2 potatoes, sliced into wedges
- 2 tablespoons olive oil, divided
- Salt and pepper to taste

- 1 red bell pepper, chopped
- ¼ cup fresh cilantro, chopped
- 1 garlic, minced
- 2 tablespoons almonds, toasted and sliced
- 1 tablespoon lime juice

Directions:

1. Warm your oven to 425 degrees F. Toss the sweet potatoes in oil and salt. Transfer to a baking pan. Roast for 20 minutes.
2. In a bowl, combine the red bell pepper, cilantro, garlic, and almonds. In another bowl, mix the lime juice, remaining oil, salt, and pepper.
3. Drizzle this mixture over the red bell pepper mixture. Serve sweet potatoes with the red bell pepper mixture.

Nutrition:

Calories: 146

Fat: 8.6g

Carbohydrates: 16g

Protein:2.3g

27. Cauliflower Salad

Preparation Time: 20 minutes

Cooking Time: 15 minutes

Servings: 4

Ingredients:

- 8 cups cauliflower florets
- 5 tablespoons olive oil, divided
- Salt and pepper to taste

- 1 cup parsley
- 1 clove garlic, minced
- 2 tablespoons lemon juice
- ¼ cup almonds, toasted and sliced
- 3 cups arugula
- 2 tablespoons olives, sliced
- ¼ cup feta, crumbled

Direction

1. Warm your oven to 425 degrees F. Toss the cauliflower in a mixture of 1 tablespoon olive oil, salt, and pepper. Place in a baking pan and roast for 15 minutes.
2. Put the parsley, remaining oil, garlic, lemon juice, salt, and pepper in a blender. Pulse until smooth. Place the roasted cauliflower in a salad bowl. Stir in the rest of the ingredients along with the parsley dressing.

Nutrition:

Calories: 198

Fat: 16.5g

Carbohydrates: 10.4g

Protein:5.4g

28. Garlic Mashed Potatoes & Turnips

Preparation Time: 20 minutes

Cooking Time: 30 minutes

Servings: 8

Ingredients:

- 1 head garlic

- 1 teaspoon olive oil
- 1 lb. turnips, sliced into cubes
- 2 lb. potatoes, sliced into cubes
- ½ cup almond milk
- ½ cup Parmesan cheese, grated
- 1 tablespoon fresh thyme, chopped
- 1 tablespoon fresh chives, chopped
- 2 tablespoons butter
- Salt and pepper to taste

Direction

1. Warm your oven to 375 degrees F. Slice the tip off the garlic head. Drizzle with a little oil and roast in the oven for 45 minutes.
2. Boil the turnips and potatoes in a pot of water for 30 minutes or until tender. Add all the ingredients to a food processor along with the garlic. Pulse until smooth. Serve.

Nutrition:

Calories: 141

Fat: 3.2g

Carbohydrates: 24.6g

Protein: 4.6g

29. Coconut Brussels Sprouts

Preparation Time: 15 minutes

Cooking Time: 10 minutes

Servings: 4

Ingredients:

- 1 lb. Brussels sprouts, trimmed and sliced in half

- 2 tablespoons coconut oil
- ¼ cup of coconut water
- 1 tablespoon soy sauce

Direction

1. Put the coconut oil in a pan over medium heat, and cook the Brussels sprouts for 4 minutes. Pour in the coconut water. Cook for 3 minutes. Add the soy sauce and cook for another 1 minute. Serve.

Nutrition:

Calories: 114

Fat: 7.1g

Carbohydrates: 11.1g

Protein: 4g

30. Stuffed Sweet Potatoes

Preparation time: 30 minutes

Cooking time: 1 hour & 16 minutes

Servings: 3

Ingredients:

- ½ cup dry black beans
- 3 small or medium sweet potatoes
- 2 tbsp. olive oil
- 1 large red bell pepper, pitted, chopped
- 1 large green bell pepper, pitted, chopped
- 1 small sweet yellow onion, chopped
- 2 tbsp. garlic, minced or powdered
- 1 8-oz. package tempeh, diced into ¼" cubes
- ½ cup marinara sauce

- ½ cup of water
- 1 tbsp chili powder
- 1 tsp. parsley
- ½ tsp. cayenne
- Salt and pepper to taste

Directions:

1. Preheat the oven to 400°F. Prick several holes in the skins of the sweet potatoes using a fork.
2. Wrap the sweet potatoes tightly with aluminum foil and place them in the oven until soft and tender, or for approximately 45 minutes.
3. While sweet potatoes are cooking, heat the olive oil in a deep pan over medium-high heat. Add the onions, bell peppers, and garlic; cook until the onions are tender, for about 10 minutes.
4. Add the water, together with the cooked beans, marinara sauce, chili powder, parsley, and cayenne. Bring the mixture to a boil and then lower the heat to medium or low.
5. Simmer for about 15 minutes until the liquid has thickened. Add the diced tempeh cubes and heat until warmed, around 1 minute. Blend in salt and pepper to taste.
6. Remove them from the oven. Slice a slit across on top of each one, but do not split the potatoes in half.
7. Top each potato with a scoop of the beans, vegetables, and tempeh mixture. Place the filled potatoes back in the hot oven for about 5 minutes. Serve after

cooling for a few minutes, or store for another day!

Nutrition:

Calories: 498

Carbs: 55.7 g

Fat: 17.1 g

Protein: 20.7 g.

31. Satay Tempeh with Cauliflower Rice

Preparation time: 60 minutes

Cooking time: 15 minutes

Servings: 4

Ingredients:

- ¼ cup of water
- 4 tbsp. peanut butter
- 3 tbsp. low sodium soy sauce
- 2 tbsp. coconut sugar
- 1 garlic clove, minced
- ½-inch ginger, minced
- 2 tsp. rice vinegar
- 1 tsp. red pepper flakes
- 4 tbsp. olive oil
- 2 8-oz. packages tempeh, drained
- 2 cups cauliflower rice
- 1 cup purple cabbage, diced
- 1 tbsp. sesame oil
- 1 tsp. agave nectar

Directions:

1. Combine the sauce fixings in a large bowl, and then whisk until the mixture is smooth and any lumps have dissolved.
2. Cut the tempeh into ½-inch cubes and put them into the sauce, stirring to make sure the cubes get coated thoroughly.
3. Put the bowl in your fridge to marinate the tempeh for up to 3 hours. Before the tempeh is done marinating, preheat the oven to 400°F.
4. Spread the tempeh out in one layer on a baking sheet lined with parchment paper or lightly greased with olive oil. Bake the marinated cubes until browned and crisp—about 15 minutes.
5. Heat the cauliflower rice in a saucepan with 2 tablespoons of olive oil over medium heat until it is warm. Rinse the large bowl with water, and then mix the cabbage, sesame oil, and agave.
6. Serve a scoop of the cauliflower rice topped with the marinated cabbage and cooked tempeh on a plate, and enjoy. Or, store for later.

Nutrition:

Calories: 531

Carbs: 31.7 g

Fat: 33 g

Protein: 27.6 g.

32. Sweet Potato Quesadillas

Preparation time: 15 minutes

Cooking time: 1 hour & 9 minutes

Servings: 3

Ingredients:

- 1 cup dry black beans
- ½ cup dry rice of choice
- 1 large sweet potato, peeled and diced
- ½ cup of salsa
- 3-6 tortilla wraps
- 1 tbsp. olive oil
- ½ tsp. garlic powder
- ½ tsp. onion powder
- ½ tsp. paprika

Directions:

1. Preheat the oven to 350°F. Line a baking pan with parchment paper. Drizzle olive oil on the sweet potato cubes. Transfer the cubes to the baking pan. Bake the potatoes in the oven until tender, for around 1 hour.
2. Allow about 5 minutes for the potatoes to cool, and then add them to a large mixing bowl with the salsa and cooked rice. Use a fork to mash the fixings into a thoroughly combined mixture.
3. Heat a saucepan over medium-high heat and add the potato/rice mixture, cooked black beans, and spices to the pan. Cook everything for about 5 minutes or until it is heated through.
4. Take another frying pan and put it over medium-low heat. Place a tortilla in the pan and fill half of it with a heaping scoop of the potato, bean, and rice mixture.
5. Fold the tortilla halfway to cover the filling and cook until both sides are browned—about 4 minutes per side.

Serve the tortillas with some additional salsa on the side.

Nutrition:

Calories: 329

Carbs: 54.8 g

Fat: 7.5 g

Protein: 10.6 g.

33. Spicy Grilled Tofu with Szechuan Vegetables

Preparation time: 5 minutes

Cooking time: 12 minutes

Servings: 2

Ingredients:

- 1 lb. firm tofu, frozen and thawed
- 3 tablespoons soy sauce
- 2 tablespoons toasted sesame oil
- 2 tablespoons apple cider vinegar
- 1 clove garlic, minced
- 1 teaspoon freshly grated ginger
- ¼ teaspoon red pepper flakes

For the vegetables:

- 1 tablespoon toasted sesame oil
- 1 lb. fresh green beans, trimmed
- 1 red bell pepper, sliced
- 1 small red onion, sliced
- 1 teaspoon soy sauce
- 2 tablespoons Szechuan sauce
- 1 teaspoon corn starch

Directions:

1. Slice your tofu into ½" slices, then place into a shallow baking dish. Take a small bowl and add the marinade ingredients. Stir well, then pour over the tofu.
2. Put in a refrigerator for at least 30 minutes. Preheat the broiler to medium, then grill the tofu until firm. Fill a pot with water and pop over medium heat.
3. Bring to the boil, then add the beans. Blanche for 2 minutes, then drain and rinse. Take a small bowl and add the corn starch and a teaspoon of cold water.
4. Place a skillet over medium heat, add the oil, then add the beans, red peppers, and onions. Stir well. Add the soy sauce and Szechuan sauce and cook for another minute.
5. Add the corn starch mixture and stir again. Serve the veggies and the tofu together.

Nutrition:

Calories: 297

Carbs: 9g

Fat: 20g

Protein: 24g

34. Vegan-Friendly Fajitas

Preparation time: 30 minutes

Cooking time: 19 minutes

Servings: 6

Ingredients:

- 1 cup dry black beans
- 1 large green bell pepper, seeded, diced
- 1 poblano pepper, seeded, thinly sliced
- 1 large avocado, peeled, pitted, mashed
- 1 medium sweet onion, chopped
- 3 large portobello mushrooms
- 2 tbsp. olive oil
- 6 tortilla wraps
- 1 tsp. lime juice
- 1 tsp. chili powder
- 1 tsp. garlic powder
- ¼ tsp. cayenne pepper
- Salt to taste

Directions:

1. Cook the black beans as recommended. Warm-up 1 tablespoon of olive oil in a large frying pan over high heat. Add the bell peppers, poblano peppers, and half of the onions.
2. Mix in the chili powder, garlic powder, and cayenne pepper; add salt to taste. Cook the vegetables until tender and browned around 10 minutes.
3. Add the black beans, continue cooking for an additional 2 minutes, then remove the frying pan from the stove.
4. Add the portobello mushrooms to the skillet and turn the heat down to low. Sprinkle the mushrooms with salt.
5. Stir/flip the ingredients often and cook until the mushrooms have shrunk to half their size, around 7 minutes. Remove the frying pan from the heat.
6. Mix the avocado, the remaining 1 tablespoon of olive oil, and the remaining onions in a small bowl to

make a simple guacamole. Stir the lime juice in and add salt and pepper to taste.

7. Spread the guacamole on a tortilla with a spoon and then top with a generous scoop of the mushroom mixture.

8. Serve and enjoy right away or prepare tortillas to cool down and wrap them in paper towels to store!

Nutrition:

Calories: 264

Carbs: 27.7 g

Fat: 14 g

Protein: 6.8 g

35. Tofu Cacciatore

Preparation time: 45 minutes

Cooking time: 35 minutes

Servings: 3

Ingredients:

- 1 14-oz. package extra-firm tofu, drained
- 1 tbsp. olive oil
- 1 cup matchstick carrots
- 1 medium sweet onion, diced
- 1 medium green bell pepper, seeded, diced
- 1 28-oz. can dice tomatoes
- 1 4-oz. can tomato paste
- ½ tbsp. balsamic vinegar
- 1 tbsp. soy sauce
- 1 tbsp. maple syrup
- 1 tbsp. garlic powder
- 1 tbsp. Italian seasoning

- Salt and pepper to taste

Directions:

1. Chop the tofu into ¼- to ½-inch cubes. Warm-up the olive oil on medium-high heat in a large skillet.

2. Add onions, garlic, bell peppers, and carrots; sauté until the onions turn translucent, around 10 minutes while stirring frequently.

3. Now add the balsamic vinegar, soy sauce, maple syrup, garlic powder, and Italian seasoning.

4. Stir well while pouring in the diced tomatoes and tomato paste; mix until all ingredients are thoroughly combined. Add the cubed tofu and stir one more time.

5. Cover the pot, turn the heat to medium-low, and allow the mixture to simmer until the sauce has thickened, for around 20-25 minutes.

6. Serve the tofu cacciatore in bowls and top with salt and pepper to taste, or store for another meal!

Nutrition:

Calories: 274

Carbs: 33.7 g

Fat: 9.5 g

Protein: 13.6 g.

36. Portobello Burritos

Preparation time: 50 minutes

Cooking time: 40 minutes

Servings: 4

Ingredients:

- 3 large portobello mushrooms
- 2 medium potatoes
- 4 tortilla wraps
- 1 medium avocado, pitted, peeled, diced
- ¾ cup of salsa
- 1 tbsp. cilantro
- ½ tsp. salt
- 1/3 cup of water
- 1 tbsp. lime juice
- 1 tbsp. minced garlic
- ¼ cup teriyaki sauce

Directions:

1. Preheat the oven to 400°F. Use olive oil to grease a sheet pan lightly (or line with parchment paper) and set it aside. Combine the water, lime juice, teriyaki, and garlic in a small bowl.
2. Slice the portobello mushrooms into thin slices and add these to the bowl. Allow the mushrooms to marinate thoroughly for up to three hours.
3. Cut the potatoes into large matchsticks, like French fries. Sprinkle the fries with salt and then transfer them to the sheet pan.
4. Place the fries in the oven and bake them until crisped and golden, around 30 minutes. Flip once halfway through for even cooking.
5. Heat a large frying pan and add the marinated mushroom slices with the remaining marinade to the pan. Cook until the liquid has absorbed, around 10 minutes. Remove from heat.
6. Fill the tortillas with a heaping scoop of the mushrooms and a handful of the potato sticks. Top with salsa, sliced avocados, and cilantro before serving.
7. Serve right away, enjoy, or store the tortillas, avocado, and mushrooms separately for later!

Nutrition:

Calories: 239

Carbs: 34 g

Fat: 9.2 g

Protein: 5.1 g.

37. Mushroom Madness Stroganoff

Preparation time: 30 minutes

Cooking time: 25 minutes

Servings: 4

Ingredients:

- 2 cups gluten-free noodles
- 1 small onion, chopped
- 2 cups vegetable broth
- 2 tbsp. almond flour
- 1 tbsp. tamari
- 1 tsp. tomato paste
- 1 tsp. lemon juice
- 3 cups mushrooms, chopped
- 1 tsp. thyme
- 3 cups raw spinach
- 1 tbsp. apple cider vinegar
- 1 tbsp. olive oil
- Salt and pepper to taste

- 2 tbsp. fresh parsley

Directions:

1. Cook the noodles, as stated in the instructions on the package. Warm-up olive oil over medium heat in a large skillet. Add the chopped onion and sauté until soft—for about 5 minutes.

2. Stir in the flour, vegetable broth, tamari, tomato paste, and lemon juice; cook for an additional 3 minutes. Blend in the mushrooms, thyme, and salt to taste, then cover the skillet.

3. Cook until the mushrooms are tender, for about 7 minutes, and turn the heat down to low. Add the cooked noodles, spinach, and vinegar to the pan and top the ingredients with salt and pepper to taste.

4. Cover the skillet again and let the flavors combine for another 8-10 minutes. Serve immediately, topped with the optional parsley if desired, or store and enjoy the stroganoff another day of the week!

Nutrition:

Calories: 200

Carbs: 27.8 g

Fat: 6.5 g

Protein: 7.6 g.

38.   Moroccan Eggplant Stew

Preparation time: 45 minutes

Cooking time: 32 minutes

Servings: 4

Ingredients:

- 1 cup dry green lentils
- 1 cup dry chickpeas
- 1 tsp. olive oil
- 1 large sweet onion, chopped
- 1 medium green bell pepper, seeded, diced
- 1 large eggplant
- 1 cup vegetable broth
- ¾ cup tomato sauce
- ½ cup golden raisins
- 2 tbsp. turmeric
- 1 garlic clove, minced
- 1 tsp. cumin
- ½ tsp. allspice
- ¼ tsp. chili powder
- Salt and pepper to taste

Directions:

1. Warm-up the olive oil in a medium skillet on medium-high heat. Add the onions and cook until they begin to caramelize and soften in 5-8 minutes.

2. Cut the eggplant into ½-inch eggplant cubes and add it to the skillet along with the bell pepper, cumin, allspice, garlic, and turmeric.

3. Stir the ingredients to combine everything evenly and heat for about 4 minutes; then add the vegetable broth and tomato sauce.

4. Cover the skillet, lower the heat, and let the ingredients simmer until the eggplant feels tender, or for about 20

minutes. You should be able to insert a fork into the cubes easily.

5. Uncover and mix in the cooked chickpeas and green lentils, as well as the raisins and chili powder. Simmer the ingredients until all the flavors have melded together, or for about 3 minutes.

6. Store the stew for later, or serve in a bowl, top with salt and pepper to taste, and enjoy!

Nutrition:

Calories: 417

Carbs: 80.5 g

Fat: 2.7 g

Protein: 17.7 g.

39. Barbecued Greens & Grits

Preparation time: 60 minutes

Cooking time: 35 minutes

Servings: 4

Ingredients:

- 1 14-oz. package tempeh, cut into slices
- 3 cups vegetable broth
- 3 cups collard greens, chopped
- ½ cup BBQ sauce
- 1 cup gluten-free grits
- ¼ cup white onion, diced
- 2 tbsp. olive oil
- 2 garlic cloves, minced
- 1 tsp. salt

Directions:

1. Preheat the oven to 400°F. Mix tempeh it with the BBQ sauce in a shallow baking dish. Set aside and let marinate for up to 3 hours. Heat 1 tbsp. Put olive oil in a frying pan, then add the garlic and sauté until fragrant.

2. Add the collard greens and ½ Teaspoon of salt and cook until the collards are wilted and dark. Remove from the heat and set aside.

3. Cover the tempeh and BBQ sauce mixture with aluminum foil—Bake in the oven the ingredients for 15 minutes. Uncover and continue to bake within another 10 minutes until the tempeh is browned and crispy.

4. While the tempeh cooks, heat the remaining tablespoon of olive oil in the previously used frying pan over medium heat. Cook the onions until brown and fragrant, around 10 minutes.

5. Put in the vegetable broth and boil; then turn the heat down to low. Slowly whisk the grits into the simmering broth. Add the remaining ½ Teaspoon of salt before covering the pan with a lid.

6. Let the ingredients simmer for about 8 minutes until the grits are soft and creamy. Serve the tempeh and collard greens on top of a bowl of grits and enjoy, or store for later!

Nutrition:

Calories: 394

Carbs: 39.3 g

Fat: 17.6 g

Protein: 19.7 g.

40. Greens and Olives Pan

Preparation time: 10 minutes

Cooking time: 15 minutes

Servings: 4

Ingredients:

- 4 spring onions, chopped
- 2 tablespoons olive oil
- ½ cup green olives pitted and halved
- ¼ cup pine nuts, toasted
- 1 tablespoon balsamic vinegar
- 2 cups baby spinach
- 1 cup baby arugula
- 1 cup asparagus, trimmed, blanched, and halved
- Salt and black pepper to the taste

Directions:

1. Heat-up a pan with the oil over medium-high heat, add the spring onions and the asparagus, and sauté for 5 minutes.
2. Add the olives, spinach, and the other ingredients, toss, cook over medium heat for 10 minutes, divide between plates and serve for lunch.

Nutrition:

Calories 136

Fat 13.1g

Carbs 4.4g

Protein 2.8g

41. Classic Black Beans Chili

Preparation time: 10 minutes

Cooking time: 3 hours

Servings: 4

Ingredients:

- ½ cup quinoa
- 2 and ½ cups veggie stock
- 14 ounces canned tomatoes, chopped
- 15 ounces canned black beans, drained
- ¼ cup green bell pepper, chopped
- ¼ cup red bell pepper, chopped
- A pinch of salt and black pepper
- 2 garlic cloves, minced
- 1 carrot, shredded
- 1 small chili pepper, chopped
- 2 teaspoons chili powder
- 1 teaspoon cumin, ground
- A pinch of cayenne pepper
- ½ cup of corn
- 1 teaspoon oregano, dried

For the vegan sour cream:

- A drizzle of apple cider vinegar
- 4 tablespoons water
- ½ cup cashews, soaked overnight and drained
- 1 teaspoon lime juice

Directions:

1. Put the stock in your slow cooker. Add quinoa, tomatoes, beans, red and green bell pepper, garlic, carrot, salt, pepper, corn, cumin, cayenne, chili powder, chili pepper oregano, stir, cover, and cook on high for 3 hours.

2. Meanwhile, put the cashews in your blender. Add water, vinegar, and lime juice and pulse well. Divide beans chili into bowls, top with vegan sour cream, and serve.

Nutrition:

Calories 300

Fat 4g

Carbs 10g

Protein 7g

42. Amazing Potato Dish

Preparation time: 10 minutes

Cooking time: 3 hours

Servings: 4

Ingredients:

- 1 and ½ pounds potatoes, peeled and roughly chopped
- 1 tablespoon olive oil
- 3 tablespoons water
- 1 small yellow onion, chopped
- ½ cup veggie stock cube, crumbled
- ½ teaspoon coriander, ground
- ½ teaspoon cumin, ground
- ½ teaspoon garam masala
- ½ teaspoon chili powder
- Black pepper to the taste
- ½ pound spinach, roughly torn

Directions:

1. Put the potatoes in your slow cooker. Add oil, water, onion, stock cube,

coriander, cumin, garam masala, chili powder, black pepper, and spinach.

2. Stir, cover, and cook on high within 3 hours. Divide into bowls and serve. Enjoy!

Nutrition:

Calories 270

Fat 4g

Carbs 8g

Protein 12g

43. Sweet Potatoes and Lentils Delight

Preparation time: 10 minutes

Cooking time: 4 hours and 30 minutes

Servings: 6

Ingredients:

- 6 cups sweet potatoes, peeled and cubed
- 2 teaspoons coriander, ground
- 2 teaspoons chili powder
- 1 yellow onion, chopped
- 3 cups veggie stock
- 4 garlic cloves, minced
- A pinch of sea salt
- black pepper
- 10 ounces canned coconut milk
- 1 cup of water
- 1 and ½ cups red lentils

Directions:

1. Put sweet potatoes in your slow cooker. Add coriander, chili powder, onion,

stock, garlic, salt, and pepper, stir, cover and cook on high for 3 hours.

2. Add lentils, stir, cover, and cook for 1 hour and 30 minutes. Add water and coconut milk, stir well, divide into bowls, and serve right away. Enjoy!

Nutrition

Calories 300

Fat 10g

Carbs 16g

Protein 10g

Chapter 3. Snack Recipes

44. Pea Dip

Preparation time: 10 minutes

Cooking time: 0 minutes

Servings: 8

Ingredients:

- 2 cups canned black-eyed peas, drained and rinsed
- ½ teaspoon chili powder
- ½ cup coconut cream
- A pinch of salt and black pepper
- ½ teaspoon garlic powder
- 1 teaspoon Italian seasoning
- ½ teaspoon chili sauce
- 1 teaspoon hot paprika

Directions:

1. In a blender, mix the peas with the chili powder, cream and the other ingredients, blend and serve.

Nutrition:

Calories 127

Fat 5g

Carbs 18g

Protein 8g

45. Chili Walnuts

Preparation time: 10 minutes

Cooking time: 10 minutes

Servings: 4

Ingredients:

- ½ teaspoon chili flakes
- ½ teaspoon curry powder
- ½ teaspoon hot paprika
- A pinch of cayenne pepper
- 14 ounces walnuts
- 2 teaspoons avocado oil

Directions:

1. Put the walnuts on your lined baking sheet, add the chili and the other ingredients, toss, introduce in the oven and bake at 400 degrees F for 10 minutes. Divide the mix into bowls and serve as a snack.

Nutrition:

Calories 204

Fat 3.2g

Carbs 7.4g

Protein 7g

46. Seed and Apricot Bowls

Preparation time: 10 minutes

Cooking time: 10 minutes

Servings: 4

Ingredients:

- 6 ounces apricots, dried
- 1 cup sunflower seeds
- 2 tablespoons coconut, shredded
- 1 tablespoon sesame seeds
- 1 tablespoon avocado oil
- 3 tablespoons hemp seeds
- 1 tablespoon chia seeds

Directions:

1. Spread the apricots, seeds and the other ingredients on a lined baking sheet, toss and cook at 430 degrees F for 10 minutes. Cool down, divide into bowls and serve as a snack.

Nutrition:

Calories 200

Fat 4.3g

Carbs 8g

Protein 5g

47. Zucchini Muffins

Preparation time: 10 minutes

Cooking time: 30 minutes

Servings: 12

Ingredients:

- 2 cups almond flour
- 2 teaspoons baking powder
- 2 tablespoons coconut sugar
- A pinch of black pepper
- 2 tbsp flaxseed meal + 3 tbsp water, mixed
- ¾ cup almond milk
- 1 cup zucchinis, grated
- ½ cup tofu, shredded

Directions:

1. In a bowl, combine the flour with baking powder, flaxseed and the other ingredients, stir well, divide into a lined muffin tray, introduce in the oven and

bake at 400 degrees F for 30 minutes. Serve as a snack.

Nutrition:

Calories 149

Fat 4g

Carbs 14g

Protein 5g

48. Nuts and Seeds Squares

Preparation Time: 20 Minutes

Cooking Time: 5 Minutes

Servings: 8

Ingredients:

- ½ cup hazelnuts, toasted
- ½ cup walnuts, toasted
- ½ cup almonds, toasted
- ½ cup white sesame seeds
- ½ cup pumpkin seeds, shelled
- 1 cup unsweetened dried cherries
- 2 cups unsweetened dried coconut flakes
- ¼ cup coconut oil
- 1/3 cup maple syrup
- ½ teaspoon ground cinnamon
- ½ teaspoon salt

Directions:

1. Prepare a 13x9-inch baking dish lined using parchment paper. Set aside. In a large bowl, add the hazelnuts, walnuts, and almonds and mix well.
2. Transfer 1 cup of the nut mixture into another large bowl and chop them

roughly. In the food processor, add the remaining nut mixture and pulse until finely ground.

3. Now, transfer the ground nut mixture into the bowl of the chopped nuts. Add the seeds and coconut flakes and mix well.

4. In a small pan, add the oil, maple syrup, and cinnamon over medium-low heat and cook for about 3–5 minutes or until it starts to boil, stirring continuously.

5. Remove from the heat and immediately pour over the nut mixture, stirring continuously until well combined. Set aside to cool slightly.

6. Now, place the mixture into the prepared baking dish evenly and with the back of a spoon, smooth the top surface by pressing slightly.

7. Refrigerate for about 1 hour or until set completely. Remove from refrigerator and cut into equal sized squares and serve.

Nutrition:

Calories: 496

Protein: 10g

Carbohydrates: 24g

Fat: 42g

49. Seed Bars

Preparation Time: 15 Minutes

Cooking Time: 15 Minutes

Servings: 10

Ingredients:

- 1¼ cups creamy salted peanut butter
- 5 Medjool dates, pitted
- ½ cup unsweetened vegan protein powder
- 2/3 cup hemp seeds
- 1/3 cup chia seeds

Directions:

1. Line a loaf pan with parchment paper. Set aside. In a food processor, add the peanut butter and dates and pulse until well combined.

2. Add the protein powder, hemp seeds, and chia seeds and pulse until well combined. Now, place the mixture into the prepared loaf pan and with the back of a spoon, smooth the top surface.

3. Freeze for at least 10–15 minutes, or until set. Cut into 10 equal sized bars and serve.

Nutrition:

Calories: 308

Fat: 21g

Carbohydrates: 17g

Protein: 16g

50. Chocolate Protein Bites

Preparation Time: 10 Minutes

Cooking Time: 20 Minutes

Servings: 12

Ingredients:

- ½ cup Chocolate Protein Powder
- 1 Avocado, medium

- 1 tbsp. Chocolate Chips
- 1 tbsp. Almond Butter
- 1 tbsp. Cocoa Powder
- 1 tsp. Vanilla Extract
- Dash of Salt

Directions:

1. Begin by blending avocado, almond butter, vanilla extract, and salt in a high-speed blender until you get a smooth mixture.
2. Next, spoon in the protein powder, cocoa powder, and chocolate chips to the blender. Blend again until you get a smooth dough-like consistency mixture.
3. Now, check for seasoning and add more sweetness if needed. Finally, with the help of a scooper, scoop out dough to make small balls.

Nutrition:

Calories: 46

Fat: 2g

Carbohydrates: 2g

Protein: 2g

51.   Spicy Nuts and Seeds Snack Mix

Preparation Time: 5 Minutes

Cooking Time: 10 Minutes

Servings: 4

Ingredients:

- ¼ tsp garlic powder
- ¼ tsp nutritional yeast
- ½ tsp smoked paprika

- ¼ tsp sea salt
- ¼ tsp dried parsley
- ½ cup slivered almonds
- ½ cup cashew pieces
- ½ cup sunflower seeds
- ½ cup pepitas

Directions:

1. Mix the garlic powder, nutritional yeast, paprika, salt, and parsley in a small bowl. Set aside. In a large skillet, add the almonds, cashews, sunflower seeds, pepitas and heat over low heat until warm and glistening, 3 minutes.
2. Turn the heat off and stir in the parsley mixture. Allow complete cooling and enjoy!

Nutrition:

Calories: 385

Fat: 33g

Protein: 12g

Carbohydrates: 16g

52.   Banana Nut Bread Bars

Preparation Time: 5 Minutes

Cooking Time: 30 Minutes

Servings: 9

Ingredients:

- Nonstick cooking spray (optional)
- 2 large ripe bananas
- 2 tablespoon maple syrup
- ½ teaspoon vanilla extract
- 2 cups old-fashioned rolled oats

- ½ teaspoons salt
- ¼ cup chopped walnuts

Directions:

1. Preheat the oven to 350ºF. Lightly coat a 9-by-9-inch baking pan with nonstick cooking spray (if using) or line with parchment paper for oil-free baking.
2. In a medium bowl, mash the bananas with a fork. Add the maple syrup and vanilla extract and mix well. Add the oats, salt, and walnuts, mixing well.
3. Move the batter to the baking pan and bake for 25 to 30 minutes, until the top is crispy. Cool completely before slicing into 9 bars. Transfer to an airtight storage container or a large plastic bag.

Nutrition:

Calories: 73

Fat: 1g

Carbohydrates: 15g

Protein: 2g

53. Rosemary and Lemon Zest Popcorn

Preparation Time: 10 Minutes

Cooking Time: 0 Minutes

Servings: 2

Ingredients:

- 1/3 cup popcorn kernels
- 2 tablespoon vegan butter, melted
- 1 tablespoon chopped rosemary
- 1 teaspoon lemon zest
- ¼ teaspoon salt

Directions:

1. Pop the kernels, and when done, transfer them into a large bowl. Drizzle butter over the popcorns, sprinkle with salt, lemon zest, and rosemary, and then toss until combined. Serve straight away.

Nutrition:

Calories: 201

Protein: 3g

Carbohydrates: 25g

Fats: 10g

54. Strawberry Avocado Toast

Preparation Time: 5 Minutes

Cooking Time: 0 Minutes

Servings: 4

Ingredients:

- 1 avocado, peeled, pitted, and quartered
- 4 whole-wheat bread slices, toasted
- 4 ripe strawberries, cut into ¼-inch slices
- 1 tablespoon balsamic glaze or reduction

Directions:

1. Mash one-quarter of your avocado on a slice of toast. Put one-quarter of the strawberry slices over your avocado, then finish with a drizzle of balsamic

glaze. Repeat with the remaining fixings, and serve.

Nutrition:

Calories: 150

Fats: 8g

Carbohydrates: 17g

Protein: 5g

55. Strawberry Watermelon Ice Pops

Preparation Time: 6 Hours & 5 Minutes

Cooking Time: 0 Minutes

Servings: 6

Ingredients:

- 4 cups diced watermelon
- 4 strawberries, tops removed
- 2 tablespoons freshly squeezed lime juice

Directions:

1. Combine the watermelon, strawberries, and lime juice in a blender. Blend within 1 to 2 minutes, or until well combined.
2. Pour evenly into 6 ice-pop molds, insert ice-pop sticks, and freeze for at least 6 hours before serving.

Nutrition:

Calories: 61

Fat: 0g

Carbohydrates: 15g

Protein: 1g

56. Carrot Energy Balls

Preparation Time: 10 Minutes

Cooking Time: 0 Minutes

Servings: 8

Ingredients:

- 1 large carrot, grated carrot
- 1 ½ cups old-fashioned oats
- 1 cup raisins
- 1 cup dates, pitied
- 1 cup coconut flakes
- 1/4 teaspoon ground cloves
- 1/2 teaspoon ground cinnamon

Directions:

1. Pulse all fixings in your food processor until it forms a sticky and uniform mixture. Shape the batter into equal balls. Place in your refrigerator until ready to serve. Bon appétit!

Nutrition:

Calories: 495

Protein: 22g

Carbohydrates: 58g

Fat: 21g

57. Sweet Potato Bites

Preparation Time: 1 hour & 10 Minutes

Cooking Time: 25 Minutes

Servings: 4

Ingredients:

- 4 sweet potatoes, peeled and grated

- 2 chia eggs
- 1/4 cup nutritional yeast
- 2 tablespoons tahini
- 2 tablespoons chickpea flour
- 1 teaspoon shallot powder
- 1 teaspoon garlic powder
- 1 teaspoon paprika
- Sea salt
- ground black pepper, to taste

Directions:

1. Warm your oven to 395 degrees F. Line a baking pan with parchment paper or Silpat mat.
2. Thoroughly combine all the ingredients until everything is well incorporated. Roll the batter into equal balls and place them in your refrigerator for about 1 hour.
3. Bake these balls for approximately 25 minutes, turning them over halfway through the cooking time. Bon appétit!

Nutrition:

Calories: 215

Fat: 4.5g

Carbohydrates: 35g

Protein: 9g

58. Banana Bulgur Bars

Preparation Time: 10 Minutes

Cooking Time: 30 Minutes

Servings: 9

Ingredients:

- 2 ripe large bananas
- 1 tablespoon pure maple syrup
- ½ teaspoon pure vanilla extract
- 1 cup rolled oats
- 1 cup medium-grind or coarse bulgur
- ¼ cup chopped walnuts

Directions:

1. Preheat the oven to 350ºF. Prepare an 8-inch square baking pan lined using parchment paper.
2. In a medium bowl, mash the bananas with a fork. Add the maple syrup and vanilla and mix well. Add the oats, bulgur, and walnuts and mix until combined.
3. Transfer the mixture to the prepared baking pan and bake for 25 to 30 minutes, until the top is crispy.
4. Let cool, then slice into 9 bars and transfer to an airtight container or a large zip-top plastic bag. Store at room temperature for up to 5 days.

Nutrition:

Calories: 142

Fat: 3g

Carbohydrates: 26g

Protein: 4g

59. Italian Tomato Snack

Preparation Time: 10 Minutes

Cooking Time: 60 Minutes

Servings: 6

Ingredients:

- 50 oz canned tomatoes, drained
- A pinch of salt and black pepper
- ¼ cup extra virgin olive oil
- 15 basil leaves, sliced
- 1 tablespoon burgundy or merlot wine vinegar
- A pinch of stevia
- 10 baguette pieces, toasted.

Directions:

1. Spread the tomatoes on the lined baking sheet, drizzle half of the oil, season with salt and pepper and bake them at 300 degrees F for one hour.
2. Slice the tomatoes into cubes, put them inside a bowl, contribute the others of the oil, basil, vinegar as well as the stevia and toss. Split the tomatoes on each baguette slice and serve as a snack.

Nutrition:

Calories: 191

Fat: 4g

Carbohydrates: 9g

Protein: 7g

60. Easy Dried Grapes

Preparation Time: 5 Minutes

Cooking Time: 4 Hours

Servings: 10

Ingredients:

- 3 bunches seedless grapes
- A drizzle of vegetable oil

Directions:

1. Spread the grapes over a lined baking sheet, drizzle the oil, toss and bake at 225 degrees F for 4 hours. Separate the grapes into bowls and serve.

Nutrition:

Calories: 131

Fat: 1g

Protein: 3g

Carbohydrates: 5g

61. Beans and Squash Dip

Preparation Time: 10 Minutes

Cooking Time: 6 Hours

Servings: 4

Ingredients:

- ½ cup butternut squash, peeled and cubed
- ½ cup canned white beans, drained
- 1 tablespoon water
- 2 tablespoons coconut milk
- ½ teaspoon rosemary, dried
- ½ teaspoon sage, dried
- A pinch of salt and black pepper

Directions:

1. In a slow cooker, mix beans with squash, water, coconut milk, sage, rosemary, salt and pepper, toss, cover and cook on Low for 6 hours. Blend using an immersion blender, divide into bowls and serve cold.

Nutrition:

Calories: 182

Fat: 5g

Carbohydrates: 12g

Protein: 4g

62. Stuffed Cherry Tomato

Preparation Time: 15 Minutes

Cooking Time: 0 Minutes

Servings: 6

Ingredients:

- 2 pints cherry tomatoes, tops removed and centers scooped out
- 2 avocados, mashed
- Juice of 1 lemon
- 1/2 red bell pepper, minced
- 4 green onions (white & green parts), finely minced
- 1 tablespoon minced fresh tarragon
- Pinch of sea salt

Directions:

1. Place the cherry tomatoes open-side up on a platter. Combine the avocado, lemon juice, bell pepper, scallions, tarragon, and salt in a small bowl.
2. Stir until well -combined. Scoop into the cherry tomatoes and serve immediately.

Nutrition:

Calories: 264

Fat: 8g

Carbohydrates: 19g

Protein: 5g

63. French Onion Pastry Puff

Preparation Time: 10 Minutes

Cooking Time: 35 Minutes

Servings: 24

Ingredients:

- 2 tablespoons olive oil
- 2 medium onions, thinly sliced
- 1 garlic clove, minced
- 1 teaspoon chopped fresh rosemary
- Salt and freshly ground black pepper
- 1 tablespoon capers
- 1 sheet frozen vegan puff pastry, thawed
- 18 pitted black olives, quartered

Directions:

1. Heat-up the oil in a medium skillet over medium heat. Add the onions and garlic, season with rosemary and salt and pepper to taste.
2. Cover and cook until very soft, stirring occasionally, about 20 minutes. Stir in the capers and set aside.
3. Preheat the oven to 400 degree F. Roll out the puff pastry and cut into 2- to 3-inch circles using a lightly floured pastry cutter or drinking glass. You should get about 2 dozen circles.
4. Arrange the pastry circles on baking sheets and top each with a heaping teaspoon of onion mixture, patting down to smooth the top.
5. Top with 3 olive quarters, arranged decoratively—either like flower petals emanating from the center or parallel to

each other like 3 bars. Bake within 15
minutes. Serve hot.

Nutrition:

Calories: 144

Protein: 5g

Carbohydrates: 18g

Fats: 7g

Chapter 4.   Salad Recipes

64.   Lebanese Potato Salad

Preparation Time: 5 minutes

Cooking Time: 10 minutes

Servings: 4

Ingredients:

- 1-pound Russet potatoes
- 1 ½ tablespoons extra virgin olive oil
- 2 scallions, thinly sliced
- Freshly ground pepper to taste
- 2 tablespoons lemon juice
- ¼ teaspoon salt or to taste
- 2 tablespoons fresh mint leaves, chopped

Directions:

1. Place a saucepan half filled with water over medium heat. Add salt and potatoes and cook for 10 minutes until tender. Drain the potatoes and place in a bowl of cold water. When cool enough to handle, peel and cube the potatoes. Place in a bowl.

To make dressing:

2. Add oil, lemon juice, salt and pepper in a bowl and whisk well. Drizzle dressing over the potatoes. Toss well.

3. Add scallions and mint and toss well.

4. Divide into 4 plates and serve.

Nutrition:

Calories 129

Total Fat 5.5g

Saturated Fat 0.9g

Cholesterol 0mg

Sodium 158mg

Total Carbohydrate 18.8g

Dietary Fiber 3.2g

Total Sugars 1.6g

Protein 2.2g

Vitamin D 0mcg

Calcium 22mg

Iron 1mg

Potassium 505mg

65.   Chickpea and Spinach Salad

Preparation Time: 5 minutes

Cooking Time: 0 minutes

Servings: 4

Ingredients:

- 2 cans (14.5 ounces each) chickpeas, drained, rinsed
- 7 ounces' vegan feta cheese, crumbled or chopped
- 1 tablespoon lemon juice
- 1/3 -½ cup olive oil
- ½ teaspoon salt or to taste
- 4-6 cups spinach, torn
- ½ cup raisins
- 2 tablespoons honey
- 1-2 teaspoons ground cumin
- 1 teaspoon chili flakes

Directions:

1. Add cheese, chickpeas and spinach into a large bowl.
2. To make dressing: Add rest of the ingredients into another bowl and mix well.
3. Pour dressing over the salad. Toss well and serve.

Nutrition:

Calories 822

Total Fat 42.5g

Saturated Fat 11.7g

Cholesterol 44mg

Sodium 910mg

Total Carbohydrate 89.6g

Dietary Fiber 19.7g

Total Sugars 32.7g

Protein 29g

Vitamin D 0mcg

Calcium 417mg

Iron 9mg

Potassium 1347mg

66.   Tempeh "Chicken" Salad

Preparation Time: 10 minutes

Cooking Time: 0 minutes

Servings: 2

Ingredients:

- 4 tablespoons light mayonnaise
- 2 scallions, sliced
- Pepper to taste
- 4 cups mixed salad greens
- 4 teaspoons white miso
- 2 tablespoons chopped fresh dill
- 1 ½ cups crumbled tempeh
- 1 cup sliced grape tomatoes

Directions:

To make dressing:

1. Add mayonnaise, scallions, miso, dill and pepper into a bowl and whisk well.
2. Add tempeh and fold gently.

To serve:

3. Divide the greens into 4 plates. Divide the tempeh among the plates. Top with tomatoes and serve.

Nutrition:

Calories 452

Total Fat 24.5g

Saturated Fat 4.4g

Cholesterol 8mg

Sodium 733mg

Total Carbohydrate 37.2g

Dietary Fiber 2.6g

Total Sugars 5.3g

Protein 29.9g

Vitamin D 0mcg

Calcium 261mg

Iron 8mg

Potassium 1377mg

67. Spinach & Dill Pasta Salad

Preparation Time: 5 minutes

Cooking Time: 0 minutes

Servings: 4

Ingredients:

For salad:

- 3 cups cooked whole-wheat fusilli
- 2 cups cherry tomatoes, halved
- ½ cup vegan cheese, shredded
- 4 cups spinach, chopped
- 2 cups edamame, thawed
- 1 large red onion, finely chopped

For dressing:

- 2 tablespoons white wine vinegar
- ½ teaspoon dried dill
- 2 tablespoons extra-virgin olive oil
- Salt to taste
- Pepper to taste

Directions:

To make dressing:

1. Add all the ingredients for dressing into a bowl and whisk well. Set aside for a while for the flavors to set in.

To make salad:

2. Add all the ingredients of the salad in a bowl. Toss well.
3. Drizzle dressing on top. Toss well.
4. Divide into 4 plates and serve.

Nutrition:

Calories 684

Total Fat 33.6g

Saturated Fat 4.6g

Cholesterol 4mg

Sodium 632mg

Total Carbohydrate 69.5g

Dietary Fiber 12g

Total Sugars 6.4g

Protein 31.7g

Vitamin D 0mcg

Calcium 368mg

Iron 8mg

Potassium 1241mg

68. Italian Veggie Salad

Preparation Time: 10 minutes

Cooking Time: 0 minutes

Servings: 8

Ingredients:

For salad:

- 1 cup fresh baby carrots, quartered lengthwise
- 1 celery rib, sliced
- 3 large mushrooms, thinly sliced
- 1 cup cauliflower florets, bite sized, blanched
- 1 cup broccoli florets, blanched
- 1 cup thinly sliced radish
- 4-5 ounces' hearts of romaine salad mix to serve

For dressing:

- ½ package Italian salad dressing mix
- 3 tablespoons white vinegar
- 3 tablespoons water
- 3 tablespoons olive oil
- 3-4 pepperoncino, chopped

Directions:

To make salad:

1. Add all the ingredients of the salad except hearts of romaine to a bowl and toss.

To make dressing:

2. Add all the ingredients of the dressing in a small bowl. Whisk well.

3. Pour dressing over salad and toss well. Refrigerate for a couple of hours.
4. Place romaine in a large bowl. Place the chilled salad over it and serve.

Nutrition:

Calories 84

Total Fat 6.7g

Saturated Fat 1.2g

Cholesterol 3mg

Sodium 212mg

Total Carbohydrate 5g

Dietary Fiber 1.4g

Total Sugars 1.6g

Protein 2g

Vitamin D 31mcg

Calcium 27mg

Iron 1mg

Potassium 193mg

69. Spinach and Mashed Tofu Salad

Preparation Time: 20 minutes

Cooking Time: 0 minutes

Servings: 4

Ingredients:

- 2 8-oz. blocks firm tofu, drained
- 4 cups baby spinach leaves
- 4 tbsp. cashew butter
- 1½ tbsp. soy sauce
- 1tbsp ginger, chopped
- 1 tsp. red miso paste
- 2 tbsp. sesame seeds
- 1 tsp. organic orange zest
- 1 tsp. nori flakes
- 2 tbsp. water

Directions:

1. Use paper towels to absorb any excess water left in the tofu before crumbling both blocks into small pieces.
2. In a large bowl, combine the mashed tofu with the spinach leaves.
3. Mix the remaining ingredients in another small bowl and, if desired, add the optional water for a smoother dressing.
4. Pour this dressing over the mashed tofu and spinach leaves.
5. Transfer the bowl to the fridge and allow the salad to chill for up to one hour. Doing so will guarantee a

better flavor. Or, the salad can be served right away. Enjoy!

Nutrition:

Calories 623

Total Fat 30.5g

Saturated Fat 5.8g

Cholesterol 0mg

Sodium 2810mg

Total Carbohydrate 48g

Dietary Fiber 5.9g

Total Sugars 3g

Protein 48.4g

Vitamin D 0mcg

Calcium 797mg

Iron 22mg

Potassium 2007mg

70. Super Summer Salad

Preparation Time: 10 minutes

Cooking Time: 0 minutes

Servings: 2

Ingredients:

Dressing:

- 1 tbsp. olive oil
- ¼ cup chopped basil
- 1 tsp. lemon juice
- ¼ tsp Salt
- 1 medium avocado, halved, diced
- ¼ cup water

Salad:

- ¼ cup dry chickpeas
- ¼ cup dry red kidney beans
- 4 cups raw kale, shredded
- 2 cups Brussel sprouts, shredded
- 2 radishes, thinly sliced
- 1 tbsp. walnuts, chopped
- 1 tsp. flax seeds
- Salt and pepper to taste

Directions:

1. Prepare the chickpeas and kidney beans according to the method.
2. Soak the flax seeds according the method, and then drain excess water.
3. Prepare the dressing by adding the olive oil, basil, lemon juice, salt, and half of the avocado to a food processor or blender, and pulse on low speed.
4. Keep adding small amounts of water until the dressing is creamy and smooth.

5. Transfer the dressing to a small bowl and set it aside.

6. Combine the kale, Brussel sprouts, cooked chickpeas, kidney beans, radishes, walnuts, and remaining avocado in a large bowl and mix thoroughly.

7. Store the mixture, or, serve with the dressing and flax seeds, and enjoy!

Nutrition:

Calories 266

Total Fat 26.6g

Saturated Fat 5.1g

Cholesterol 0mg

Sodium 298mg

Total Carbohydrate 8.8g

Dietary Fiber 6.8g

Total Sugars 0.6g

Protein 2g

Vitamin D 0mcg

Calcium 19mg

Iron 1mg

Potassium 500mg

71. Roasted Almond Protein Salad

Preparation Time: 30 minutes

Cooking Time: 0 minutes

Servings: 4

Ingredients:

- ½ cup dry quinoa
- ½ cup dry navy beans
- ½ cup dry chickpeas
- ½ cup raw whole almonds
- 1 tsp. extra virgin olive oil
- ½ tsp. salt
- ½ tsp. paprika
- ½ tsp. cayenne
- Dash of chili powder
- 4 cups spinach, fresh or frozen
- ¼ cup purple onion, chopped

Directions:

1. Prepare the quinoa according to the recipe. Store in the fridge for now.

2. Prepare the beans according to the method. Store in the fridge for now.

3. Toss the almonds, olive oil, salt, and spices in a large bowl, and stir until the ingredients are evenly coated.

4. Put a skillet over medium-high heat, and transfer the almond mixture to the heated skillet.

5. Roast while stirring until the almonds are browned, around 5 minutes. You may hear the ingredients pop and crackle in the pan as they warm up. Stir frequently to prevent burning.

6. Turn off the heat and toss the cooked and chilled quinoa and beans, onions, spinach, or mixed greens in the skillet. Stir well before transferring the roasted almond salad to a bowl.

7. Enjoy the salad with a dressing of choice, or, store for later!

Nutrition:

Calories 347

Total Fat 10.5g

Saturated Fat 1g

Cholesterol 0mg

Sodium 324mg

Total Carbohydrate 49.2g

Dietary Fiber 14.7g

Total Sugars 4.7g

Protein 17.2g

Vitamin D 0mcg

Calcium 139mg

Iron 5mg

Potassium 924mg

72. Lentil, Lemon & Mushroom Salad

Preparation Time: 10 minutes

Cooking Time: 0 minutes

Servings: 2

Ingredients:

- ½ cup dry lentils of choice
- 2 cups vegetable broth
- 3 cups mushrooms, thickly sliced
- 1 cup sweet or purple onion, chopped
- 4 tsp. extra virgin olive oil
- 2 tbsp. garlic powder
- ¼ tsp. chili flakes
- 1 tbsp. lemon juice
- 2 tbsp. cilantro, chopped
- ½ cup arugula
- ¼ tsp Salt
- ¼ tsp pepper

Directions:

1. Sprout the lentils according the method. (Don't cook them).
2. Place the vegetable stock in a deep saucepan and bring it to a boil.

3. Add the lentils to the boiling broth, cover the pan, and cook for about 5 minutes over low heat until the lentils are a bit tender.
4. Remove the pan from heat and drain the excess water.
5. Put a frying pan over high heat and add 2 tablespoons of olive oil.
6. Add the onions, garlic, and chili flakes, and cook until the onions are almost translucent, around 5 to 10 minutes while stirring.
7. Add the mushrooms to the frying pan and mix in thoroughly. Continue cooking until the onions are completely translucent and the mushrooms have softened; remove the pan from the heat.
8. Mix the lentils, onions, mushrooms, and garlic in a large bowl.
9. Add the lemon juice and the remaining olive oil. Toss or stir to combine everything thoroughly.
10. Serve the mushroom/onion mixture over some arugala in bowl, adding salt and pepper to taste, or, store and enjoy later!

Nutrition:

Calories 365

Total Fat 11.7g

Saturated Fat 1.9g

Cholesterol 0mg

Sodium 1071mg

Total Carbohydrate 45.2g

Dietary Fiber 18g

Total Sugars 8.2g

Protein 22.8g

Vitamin D 378mcg

Calcium 67mg

Iron 8mg

Potassium 1212mg

73. Sweet Potato & Black Bean Protein Salad

Preparation Time: 15 minutes

Cooking Time: 0 minutes

Servings: 2

Ingredients:

- 1 cup dry black beans
- 4 cups of spinach
- 1 medium sweet potato
- 1 cup purple onion, chopped
- 2 tbsp. olive oil
- 2 tbsp. lime juice
- 1 tbsp. minced garlic

- ½ tbsp. chili powder
- ¼ tsp. cayenne
- ¼ cup parsley
- ¼ tsp Salt
- ¼ tsp pepper

Directions:

1. Prepare the black beans according to the method.
2. Preheat the oven to 400°F.
3. Cut the sweet potato into ¼-inch cubes and put these in a medium-sized bowl. Add the onions, 1 tablespoon of olive oil, and salt to taste.
4. Toss the ingredients until the sweet potatoes and onions are completely coated.
5. Transfer the ingredients to a baking sheet lined with parchment paper and spread them out in a single layer.
6. Put the baking sheet in the oven and roast until the sweet potatoes start to turn brown and crispy, around 40 minutes.
7. Meanwhile, combine the remaining olive oil, lime juice, garlic, chili powder, and cayenne thoroughly in a large bowl, until no lumps remain.
8. Remove the sweet potatoes and onions from the oven and transfer them to the large bowl.
9. Add the cooked black beans, parsley, and a pinch of salt.
10. Toss everything until well combined.
11. Then mix in the spinach, and serve in desired portions with additional salt and pepper.
12. Store or enjoy!

Nutrition:

Calories 558

Total Fat 16.2g

Saturated Fat 2.5g

Cholesterol 0mg

Sodium 390mg

Total Carbohydrate 84g

Dietary Fiber 20.4g

Total Sugars 8.9g

Protein 25.3g

Vitamin D 0mcg

Calcium 220mg

Iron 10mg

Potassium 2243mg

74. Lentil Radish Salad

Preparation Time: 15 minutes

Cooking Time: 0 minutes

Servings: 3

Ingredients:

Dressing:

- 1 tbsp. extra virgin olive oil
- 1 tbsp. lemon juice
- 1 tbsp. maple syrup
- 1 tbsp. water
- ½ tbsp. sesame oil
- 1 tbsp. miso paste, yellow or white
- ¼ tsp. salt
- ¼ tsp Pepper

Salad:

- ½ cup dry chickpeas
- ¼ cup dry green or brown lentils
- 1 14-oz. pack of silken tofu
- 5 cups mixed greens, fresh or frozen
- 2 radishes, thinly sliced
- ½ cup cherry tomatoes, halved
- ¼ cup roasted sesame seeds

Directions:

1. Prepare the chickpeas according to the method.
2. Prepare the lentils according to the method.
3. Put all the ingredients for the dressing in a blender or food processor. Mix on low until smooth, while adding water until it reaches the desired consistency.
4. Add salt, pepper (to taste), and optionally more water to the dressing; set aside.
5. Cut the tofu into bite-sized cubes.
6. Combine the mixed greens, tofu, lentils, chickpeas, radishes, and tomatoes in a large bowl.
7. Add the dressing and mix everything until it is coated evenly.
8. Top with the optional roasted sesame seeds, if desired.
9. Refrigerate before serving and enjoy, or, store for later!

Nutrition:

Calories 621

Total Fat 19.6g

Saturated Fat 2.8g

Cholesterol 0mg

Sodium 996mg

Total Carbohydrate 82.7g

Dietary Fiber 26.1g

Total Sugars 20.7g

Protein 31.3g

Vitamin D 0mcg

Calcium 289mg

Iron 9mg

Potassium 1370mg

75. Jicama and Spinach Salad Recipe

Preparation Time: 10 minutes

Cooking Time: 20 minutes

Servings: 4

Ingredients:

Salad:

- 10 oz baby spinach, washed and dried
- Grape or cherry tomatoes, cut in half
- 1 jicama, washed, peeled, and cut in strips
- Green or Kalamata olives, chopped
- 8 tsp walnuts, chopped
- 1 tsp raw or roasted sunflower seeds
- Maple Mustard Dressing

Dressing:

- 1 heaping tbsp Dijon mustard
- Dash cayenne pepper
- 2 tbsp maple syrup
- 2 garlic cloves, minced
- 1 to 2 tbsp water
- ¼ tsp sea salt

Directions:

For the salad:

1. Divide the baby spinach onto 4 salad plates. Top each serving with ¼ of the jicama, ¼ of the chopped olives, and 4 tomatoes. Sprinkle 1 tsp of the sunflower seeds and 2 tsp of the walnuts.

For the dressing:

2. In a small mixing bowl, whisk all the ingredients together until emulsified. Check the taste and add more maple syrup for sweetness.
3. Drizzle 1½ tbsp of the dressing over each salad and serve.

Nutrition:

Calories: 196

Fat: 2 g

Protein: 7 g

Carbs: 28 g

Fiber: 12g

76. High-Protein Salad

Preparation Time: 5 minutes

Cooking Time: 5 minutes

Servings: 4

Ingredients:

Salad:

- 1 15-oz can green kidney beans
- 2 4 tbsp capers
- 3 4 handfuls arugula
- 4 15-oz can lentils

  Dressing:
- 5 1 tbsp caper brine
- 6 1 tbsp tamari
- 7 1 tbsp balsamic vinegar
- 8 2 tbsp peanut butter
- 9 2 tbsp hot sauce
- 10 1 tbsp tahini

Directions:

1. For the dressing:
2. In a bowl, whisk together all the ingredients until they come together to form a smooth dressing.
3. For the salad:
4. Mix the beans, arugula, capers, and lentils. Top with the dressing and serve.

Nutrition:

Calories: 205

Fat: 2 g

Protein: 13 g

Carbs: 31 g

Fiber: 17g

Chapter 5.　　Soup and Stews Recipes

77.　Spinach Soup with Dill and Basil

Preparation Time: 10 minutes

Cooking Time: 25 minutes

Servings: 8

Ingredients:

- 1 pound peeled and diced potatoes
- 1 tablespoon minced garlic
- 1 teaspoon dry mustard
- 6 cups vegetable broth
- 20 ounces chopped frozen spinach
- 2 cups chopped onion
- 1 ½ tablespoons salt
- ½ cup minced dill
- 1 cup basil
- ½ teaspoon ground black pepper

Directions:

1. Whisk onion, garlic, potatoes, broth, mustard, and salt in a pan and cook it over medium flame. When it starts boiling, low down the heat and cover it with the lid and cook for 20 minutes.
2. Add the remaining ingredients in it and blend it and cook it for few more minutes and serve it.

Nutrition:

Carbohydrates 12g

protein 13g

fats 1g

calories 165.

78.　Coconut Watercress Soup

Preparation Time: 10 minutes

Cooking Time: 20 minutes

Servings: 4

Ingredients:

- 1 teaspoon coconut oil
- 1 onion, diced
- ¾ cup coconut milk

Directions:

Preparing the ingredients.

1. Melt the coconut oil in a large pot over medium-high heat. Add the onion and cook until soft, about 5 minutes, then add the peas and the water. Bring to a boil, lower the heat and add the watercress, mint, salt, and pepper.
2. Cover and simmer for 5 minutes. Stir in the coconut milk, and purée the soup until smooth in a blender or with an immersion blender.

3. Try this soup with any other fresh, leafy green—anything from spinach to collard greens to arugula to swiss chard.

Nutrition:

Calories: 160 kcal

Fat: 5g

Carbs: 25g

Proteins: 2g

79. Roasted Red Pepper and Butternut Squash Soup

Preparation Time: 10 minutes

Cooking Time: 45 minutes

Servings: 6

Ingredients:

- 1 small butternut squash
- 1 tablespoon olive oil
- 1 teaspoon sea salt
- 2 red bell peppers
- 1 yellow onion
- 1 head garlic
- 2 cups water, or vegetable broth
- Zest and juice of 1 lime
- 1 to 2 tablespoons tahini
- Pinch cayenne pepper
- ½ teaspoon ground coriander
- ½ teaspoon ground cumin

- Toasted squash seeds (optional)

Directions:

1. Preparing the ingredients.
2. Preheat the oven to 350°f.
3. Prepare the squash for roasting by cutting it in half lengthwise, scooping out the seeds, and poking holes in the flesh with a fork. Reserve the seeds if desired.
4. Rub a small amount of oil over the flesh and skin, rub with a bit of sea salt and put the halves skin-side down in a large baking dish. Put it in the oven while you prepare the rest of the vegetables.
5. Prepare the peppers the same way, except they do not need to be poked.
6. Slice the onion in half and rub oil on the exposed faces. Slice the top off the head of garlic and rub oil on the exposed flesh.
7. After the squash has cooked for 20 minutes, add the peppers, onion, and garlic, and roast for another 20 minutes. Optionally, you can toast the squash seeds by putting them in the oven in a separate baking dish 10 to 15 minutes before the vegetables are finished.
8. Keep a close eye on them. When the vegetables are cooked, take them out

and let them cool before handling them. The squash will be very soft when poked with a fork.

9. Scoop the flesh out of the squash skin into a large pot (if you have an immersion blender) or into a blender.

10. Chop the pepper roughly, remove the onion skin and chop the onion roughly, and squeeze the garlic cloves out of the head, all into the pot or blender. Add the water, the lime zest and juice, and the tahini. Purée the soup, adding more water if you like, to your desired consistency. Season with the salt, cayenne, coriander, and cumin. Serve garnished with toasted squash seeds (if using).

Nutrition:

calories: 156

protein: 4g

total fat: 7g

saturated fat: 11g

carbohydrates: 22g

fiber: 5g

80.   Cauliflower Spinach Soup

Preparation Time: 30 minutes

Cooking Time: 25 minutes

Servings: 5

Ingredients:

- 1/2 cup unsweetened coconut milk
- 5 oz fresh spinach, chopped
- 5 watercress, chopped
- 8 cups vegetable stock
- 1 lb cauliflower, chopped
- Salt

Directions:

1. Add stock and cauliflower in a large saucepan and bring to boil over medium heat for 15 minutes.
2. Add spinach and watercress and cook for another 10 minutes.
3. Remove from heat and puree the soup using a blender until smooth.
4. Add coconut milk and stir well. Season with salt.
5. Stir well and serve hot.

Nutrition:

Calories: 271 kcal

Fat: 3.7g

Carbs: 54g

Proteins: 6.5g

81.   Avocado Mint Soup

Preparation Time: 10 minutes

Cooking Time: 10 minutes

Servings: 2

Ingredients:

- 1 medium avocado, peeled, pitted, and cut into pieces
- 1 cup coconut milk
- 2 romaine lettuce leaves
- 20 fresh mint leaves
- 1 tbsp fresh lime juice
- 1/8 tsp salt

Directions:

1. Add all ingredients into the blender and blend until smooth. Soup should be thick not as a puree.
2. Pour into the serving bowls and place in the refrigerator for 10 minutes.
3. Stir well and serve chilled.

Nutrition:

Calories: 377 kcal

Fat: 14.9g

Carbs: 60.7g

Protein: 6.4g

82. Creamy Squash Soup

Preparation Time: 10 minutes

Cooking Time: 25 minutes

Servings: 8

Ingredients:

- 3 cups butternut squash, chopped
- 1 ½ cups unsweetened coconut milk
- 1 tbsp coconut oil
- 1 tsp dried onion flakes
- 1 tbsp curry powder
- 4 cups water
- 1 garlic clove
- 1 tsp kosher salt

Directions:

1. Add squash, coconut oil, onion flakes, curry powder, water, garlic, and salt into a large saucepan. Bring to boil over high heat.
2. Turn heat to medium and simmer for 20 minutes.
3. Puree the soup using a blender until smooth. Return soup to the saucepan and stir in coconut milk and cook for 2 minutes.
4. Stir well and serve hot.

Nutrition:

Calories: 271 kcal

Fat: 3.7g

Carbs: 54g

Protein:6.5g

83. Zucchini Soup

Preparation Time: 10 minutes

Cooking Time: 15 minutes

Servings: 8

Ingredients:

- 2 ½ lbs zucchini, peeled and sliced
- 1/3 cup basil leaves
- 4 cups vegetable stock
- 4 garlic cloves, chopped
- 2 tbsp olive oil
- 1 medium onion, diced
- Pepper
- Salt

Directions:

1. Heat olive oil in a pan over medium-low heat.
2. Add zucchini and onion and sauté until softened. Add garlic and sauté for a minute.
3. Add vegetable stock and simmer for 15 minutes.
4. Remove from heat. Stir in basil and puree the soup using a blender until smooth and creamy. Season with pepper and salt.
5. Stir well and serve.

Nutrition:

Calories: 434 kcal

Fat: 35g

Carbs: 27g

Protein: 6.7g

84. Creamy Celery Soup

Preparation Time: 20 minutes

Cooking Time: 20 minutes

Servings: 4

Ingredients:

- 6 cups celery
- ½ tsp dill
- 2 cups water
- 1 cup coconut milk
- 1 onion, chopped
- Pinch of salt

Directions:

1. Add all ingredients into the electric pot and stir well.
2. Cover electric pot with the lid and select soup setting.
3. Release pressure using a quick release method than open the lid.
4. Puree the soup using an immersion blender until smooth and creamy.
5. Stir well and serve warm.

Nutrition:

Calories: 159kcal

Fat: 8.4g

Carbs: 19.8g

Proteins: 4.6g

85.   Avocado Cucumber Soup

Preparation Time: 20 minutes

Cooking Time: 0 minutes

Servings: 3

Ingredients:

- 1 large cucumber, peeled and sliced
- ¾ cup water
- ¼ cup lemon juice
- 2 garlic cloves
- 6 green onion
- 2 avocados, pitted
- ½ tsp black pepper
- ½ tsp pink salt

Directions:

1. Add all ingredients into the blender and blend until smooth and creamy.
2. Place in refrigerator for 30 minutes.
3. Stir well and serve chilled.

Nutrition:

Calories: 127 kcal

Fat: 6.6g

Carbs: 13g

Protein: 0.7g

86.   Garden Vegetable Stew

Preparation Time: 5 minutes

Cooking Time: 60 minutes

Servings: 4

Ingredients:

- 2 tablespoons olive oil
- 1 medium red onion, chopped
- 1 medium carrot, cut into 1/4-inch slices
- 1/2 cup dry white wine
- 3 medium new potatoes, unpeeled and cut into 1-inch pieces
- 1 medium red bell pepper, cut into 1/2-inch dice
- 11/2 cups vegetable broth
- 1 tablespoon minced fresh savory or 1 teaspoon dried

Directions:

1. In a large saucepan, heat the oil over medium heat. Add the onion and carrot, cover, and cook until softened, 7 minutes. Add the wine and cook, uncovered, for 5 minutes. Stir in the potatoes, bell pepper, and broth and

bring to a boil. Reduce the heat to medium and simmer for 15 minutes.

2. Add the zucchini, yellow squash, and tomatoes. Season with salt and black pepper to taste, cover, and simmer until the vegetables are tender, 20 to 30 minutes. Stir in the corn, peas, basil, parsley, and savory. Taste, adjusting seasonings if necessary. Simmer to blend flavors, about 10 minutes more. Serve immediately.

Nutrition:

Calories: 219 kcal

Fat: 4.5g

Carbs: 38.2g

Protein: 6.4g

87. Moroccan Vermicelli Vegetable Soup

Preparation Time: 5 minutes

Cooking Time: 35 minutes

Servings: 4 to 6

Ingredients:

- 1 tablespoon olive oil
- 1 small onion, chopped
- 1 large carrot, chopped
- 1 celery rib, chopped

- 3 small zucchinis, cut into 1/4-inch dice
- 1 (28-ounce) can diced tomatoes, drained
- 2 tablespoons tomato paste
- 11/2 cups cooked or 1 (15.5-ounce) can chickpeas, drained and rinsed
- 2 teaspoons smoked paprika
- 1 teaspoon ground cumin
- 1 teaspoon za'atar spice (optional)
- 1/4 teaspoon ground cayenne
- 6 cups vegetable broth, homemade (see light vegetable broth) or store-bought, or water
- Salt
- 4 ounces' vermicelli
- 2 tablespoons minced fresh cilantro, for garnish

Directions:

1. In a large soup pot, heat the oil over medium heat. Add the onion, carrot, and celery. Cover and cook until softened, about 5 minutes. Stir in the zucchini, tomatoes, tomato paste, chickpeas, paprika, cumin, za'atar, and cayenne.

2. Add the broth and salt to taste. Bring to a boil, then reduce heat to low and simmer, uncovered, until the vegetables are tender, about 30 minutes.

3. Shortly before serving, stir in the vermicelli and cook until the noodles

are tender, about 5 minutes. Ladle the soup into bowls, garnish with cilantro, and serve.

Nutrition:

Calories: 236 kcal

Fat: 1.8g

Carbs: 48.3g

Protein: 7g

88. Moroccan Vegetable Stew

Preparation Time: 5 minutes

Cooking Time: 35 minutes

Servings: 4

Ingredients:

- 1 tablespoon olive oil
- 2 medium yellow onions, chopped
- 2 medium carrots, cut into 1/2-inch dice
- 1/2 teaspoon ground cumin
- 1/2 teaspoon ground cinnamon or allspice
- 1/2 teaspoon ground ginger
- 1/2 teaspoon sweet or smoked paprika
- 1/2 teaspoon saffron or turmeric
- 1 (14.5-ounce) can diced tomatoes, undrained
- 8 ounces' green beans, trimmed and cut into 1-inch pieces
- 2 cups peeled, seeded, and diced winter squash
- 1 large russet or other baking potato, peeled and cut into 1/2-inch dice
- 11/2 cups vegetable broth
- 11/2 cups cooked or 1 (15.5-ounce) can chickpeas, drained and rinsed
- ¾ cup frozen peas
- 1/2 cup pitted dried plums (prunes)
- 1 teaspoon lemon zest
- Salt and freshly ground black pepper
- 1/2 cup pitted green olives
- 1 tablespoon minced fresh cilantro or parsley, for garnish
- 1/2 cup toasted slivered almonds, for garnish

Directions:

1. In a large saucepan, heat the oil over medium heat. Add the onions and carrots, cover, and cook for 5 minutes. Stir in the cumin, cinnamon, ginger, paprika, and saffron. Cook, uncovered, stirring, for 30 seconds.

2. Add the tomatoes, green beans, squash, potato, and broth and bring to a boil. Reduce heat to low, cover, and simmer until the vegetables are tender, about 20 minutes.

3. Add the chickpeas, peas, dried plums, and lemon zest. Season with salt and

pepper to taste. Stir in the olives and simmer, uncovered, until the flavors are blended, about 10 minutes. Sprinkle with cilantro and almonds and serve immediately.

Nutrition:

Calories: 71 kcal

Fat: 2.8g

Carbs: 9.8g

Protein: 3.7g

89. Basic Recipe for Vegetable Broth

Preparation Time: 10 Minutes

Cooking Time: 60 Minutes

Servings: Makes 2 Quarts

Ingredients:

- 8 cups Water
- 1 Onion, chopped
- 4 Garlic cloves, crushed
- 2 Celery Stalks, chopped
- Pinch of Salt
- 1 Carrot, chopped
- Dash of Pepper
- 1 Potato, medium & chopped
- 1 tbsp. Soy Sauce
- 3 Bay Leaves

Directions:

1. To make the vegetable broth, you need to place all of the ingredients in a deep saucepan.
2. Heat the pan over a medium-high heat. Bring the vegetable mixture to a boil.
3. Once it starts boiling, lower the heat to medium-low and allow it to simmer for at least an hour or so. Cover it with a lid.
4. When the time is up, pass it through a filter and strain the vegetables, garlic, and bay leaves.
5. Allow the stock to cool completely and store in an air-tight container.

Nutrition:

Calories: 44 kcal

Fat: 0.6g

Carbs: 9.7g

Protein: 0.9g

90. Cucumber Dill Gazpacho

Preparation Time: 10 Minutes

Cooking Time: 2 hours

Serving Size: 4

Ingredients:

- 4 large cucumbers, peeled, deseeded, and chopped
- 1/8 tsp salt
- 1 tsp chopped fresh dill + more for garnishing
- 2 tbsp freshly squeezed lemon juice
- 1 ½ cups green grape, seeds removed
- 3 tbsp extra virgin olive oil
- 1 garlic clove, minced

Directions:

1. Add all the ingredients to a food processor and blend until smooth.
2. Pour the soup into serving bowls and chill for 1 to 2 hours.
3. Garnish with dill and serve chilled.

Nutrition:

Calories: 236 kcal

Fat: 1.8g

Carbs: 48.3g

Protein: 7g

Chapter 6.   Smoothie and Juices recipes

91.   Kale Smoothie

Preparation Time: 5 minutes

Cooking Time: 0 minutes

Servings: 2

Ingredients:

- 2 cups chopped kale leaves
- 1 banana, peeled
- 1 cup frozen strawberries
- 1 cup unsweetened almond milk
- 4 Medjool dates, pitted and chopped

Directions:

1. Put all the ingredients in a food processor, then blitz until glossy and smooth.
2. Serve immediately or chill in the refrigerator for an hour before serving.

Nutrition:

calories: 663

fat: 10.0g

carbs: 142.5g

fiber: 19.0g

protein: 17.4g

92.   Hot Tropical Smoothie

Preparation Time: 5 minutes

Cooking Time: 0 minutes

Servings: 4

Ingredients:

- 1 cup frozen mango chunks
- 1 cup frozen pineapple chunks
- 1 small tangerine, peeled and pitted
- 2 cups spinach leaves
- 1 cup coconut water
- ¼ teaspoon cayenne pepper, optional

Directions:

1. Add all the ingredients in a food processor, then blitz until the mixture is smooth and combine well.
2. Serve immediately or chill in the refrigerator for an hour before serving.

Nutrition:

calories: 283

fat: 1.9g

carbs: 67.9g

fiber: 10.4g

protein: 6.4g

93. Berry Smoothie

Preparation Time: 5 minutes

Cooking Time: 0 minutes

Servings: 4

Ingredients:

- 1 cup berry mix (strawberries, blueberries, and cranberries)
- 4 Medjool dates, pitted and chopped
- 1½ cups unsweetened almond milk, plus more as needed

Directions:

1. Add all the ingredients in a blender, then process until the mixture is smooth and well mixed.
2. Serve immediately or chill in the refrigerator for an hour before serving.

Nutrition:

calories: 473

fat: 4.0g

carbs: 103.7g

fiber: 9.7g

protein: 14.8g

94. Cranberry and Banana Smoothie

Preparation Time: 5 minutes

Cooking Time: 0 minutes

Servings: 4

- 1 cup frozen cranberries
- 1 large banana, peeled
- 4 Medjool dates, pitted and chopped
- 1½ cups unsweetened almond milk

Directions:

1. Add all the ingredients in a food processor, then process until the mixture is glossy and well mixed.
2. Serve immediately or chill in the refrigerator for an hour before serving.

Nutrition:

calories: 616

fat: 8.0g

carbs: 132.8g

fiber: 14.6g

protein: 15.7g

95. Pumpkin Smoothie

Preparation Time: 5 minutes

Cooking Time: 0 minutes

Servings: 5

Ingredients:

- ½ cup pumpkin purée
- 4 Medjool dates, pitted and chopped
- 1 cup unsweetened almond milk
- ¼ teaspoon vanilla extract
- ¼ teaspoon ground cinnamon
- ½ cup ice
- Pinch ground nutmeg

Directions:

1. Add all the ingredients in a blender, then process until the mixture is glossy and well mixed.
2. Serve immediately.

Nutrition:

calories: 417

fat: 3.0g

carbs: 94.9g

fiber: 10.4g

protein: 11.4g

96. Super Smoothie

Preparation Time: 5 minutes

Cooking Time: 0 minutes

Servings: 4

Ingredients:

- 1 banana, peeled
- 1 cup chopped mango
- 1 cup raspberries
- ¼ cup rolled oats
- 1 carrot, peeled
- 1 cup chopped fresh kale
- 2 tablespoons chopped fresh parsley
- 1 tablespoon flaxseeds
- 1 tablespoon grated fresh ginger
- ½ cup unsweetened soy milk
- 1 cup water

Directions:

1. Put all the ingredients in a food processor, then blitz until glossy and smooth.
2. Serve immediately or chill in the refrigerator for an hour before serving.

Nutrition:

calories: 550

fat: 39.0g

carbs: 31.0g

fiber: 15.0g

protein: 13.0g

97. Kiwi and Strawberry Smoothie

Preparation Time: 5 minutes

Cooking Time: 0 minutes

Servings: 3

Ingredients:

- 1 kiwi, peeled
- 5 medium strawberries
- ½ frozen banana
- 1 cup unsweetened almond milk
- 2 tablespoons hemp seeds
- 2 tablespoons peanut butter
- 1 to 2 teaspoons maple syrup
- ½ cup spinach leaves
- Handful broccoli sprouts

Directions:

1. Put all the ingredients in a food processor, then blitz until creamy and smooth.
2. Serve immediately or chill in the refrigerator for an hour before serving.

Nutrition:

calories: 562

fat: 28.6g

carbs: 63.6g

fiber: 15.1g

protein: 23.3g

98. Banana and Chai Chia Smoothie

Preparation Time: 5 minutes

Cooking Time: 0 minutes

Servings: 3

Ingredients:

- 1 banana
- 1 cup alfalfa sprouts
- 1 tablespoon chia seeds
- ½ cup unsweetened coconut milk
- 1 to 2 soft Medjool dates, pitted
- ¼ teaspoon ground cinnamon
- 1 tablespoon grated fresh ginger
- 1 cup water
- Pinch ground cardamom

Directions:

1. Add all the ingredients in a blender, then process until the mixture is smooth and creamy. Add water or coconut milk if necessary.
2. Serve immediately.

Nutrition:

calories: 477

fat: 41.0g

carbs: 31.0g

fiber: 14.0g

protein: 8.0g

99. Chocolate and Peanut Butter Smoothie

Preparation Time: 5 minutes

Cooking Time: 0 minutes

Servings: 4

Ingredients:

- 1 tablespoon unsweetened cocoa powder
- 1 tablespoon peanut butter
- 1 banana
- 1 teaspoon maca powder
- ½ cup unsweetened soy milk
- ¼ cup rolled oats
- 1 tablespoon flaxseeds
- 1 tablespoon maple syrup
- 1 cup water

Directions:

1. Add all the ingredients in a blender, then process until the mixture is smooth and creamy. Add water or soy milk if necessary.
2. Serve immediately.

Nutrition:

calories: 474

fat: 16.0g

carbs: 27.0g

fiber: 18.0g

protein: 13.0g

100. Golden Milk

Preparation Time: 5 minutes

Cooking Time: 0 minutes

Servings: 4

Ingredients:

- ¼ teaspoon ground cinnamon
- ½ teaspoon ground turmeric
- ½ teaspoon grated fresh ginger
- 1 teaspoon maple syrup
- 1 cup unsweetened coconut milk
- Ground black pepper, to taste
- 2 tablespoon water

Directions:

1. Combine all the ingredients in a saucepan. Stir to mix well.
2. Heat over medium heat for 5 minutes. Keep stirring during the heating.
3. Allow to cool for 5 minutes, then pour the mixture in a blender. Pulse until creamy and smooth. Serve immediately.

Nutrition:

calories: 577

fat: 57.3g

carbs: 19.7g

fiber: 6.1g

protein: 5.7g

101. Mango Agua Fresca

Preparation Time: 5 minutes

Cooking Time: 0 minutes

Servings: 2

Ingredients:

- 2 fresh mangoes, diced
- 1½ cups water
- 1 teaspoon fresh lime juice
- Maple syrup, to taste
- 2 cups ice
- 2 slices fresh lime, for garnish
- 2 fresh mint sprigs, for garnish

Directions:

1. Put the mangoes, lime juice, maple syrup, and water in a blender. Process until creamy and smooth.
2. Divide the beverage into two glasses, then garnish each glass

with ice, lime slice, and mint sprig before serving.

Nutrition:

calories: 230

fat: 1.3g

carbs: 57.7g

fiber: 5.4g

protein: 2.8g

102. Light Ginger Tea

Preparation Time: 5 minutes

Cooking Time: 10 to 15 minutes

Servings: 2

Ingredients:

- 1 small ginger knob, sliced into four 1-inch chunks
- 4 cups water
- Juice of 1 large lemon
- Maple syrup, to taste

Directions:

1. Add the ginger knob and water in a saucepan, then simmer over medium heat for 10 to 15 minutes.
2. Turn off the heat, then mix in the lemon juice. Strain the liquid to

remove the ginger, then fold in the maple syrup and serve.

Nutrition:

calories: 32

fat: 0.1g

carbs: 8.6g

fiber: 0.1g

protein: 0.1g

103. Classic Switchel

Preparation Time: 5 minutes

Cooking Time: 0 minutes

Servings: 4

Ingredients:

- 1-inch piece ginger, minced
- 2 tablespoons apple cider vinegar
- 2 tablespoons maple syrup
- 4 cups water
- ¼ teaspoon sea salt, optional

Directions:

1. Combine all the ingredients in a glass. Stir to mix well.
2. Serve immediately or chill in the refrigerator for an hour before serving.

Nutrition:

calories: 110

fat: 0g

carbs: 28.0g

fiber: 0g

protein: 0g

104. Lime and Cucumber Electrolyte Drink

Preparation Time: 5 minutes

Cooking Time: 0 minutes

Servings: 4

Ingredients:

- ¼ cup chopped cucumber
- 1 tablespoon fresh lime juice
- 1 tablespoon apple cider vinegar
- 2 tablespoons maple syrup
- ¼ teaspoon sea salt, optional
- 4 cups water

Directions:

1. Combine all the ingredients in a glass. Stir to mix well.
2. Refrigerate overnight before serving.

Nutrition:

calories: 114

fat: 0.1g

carbs: 28.9g

fiber: 0.3g

protein: 0.3g

Chapter 7.   Dinners Recipes

105. Broccoli and Rice Stir Fry

Preparation time: 5 minutes

Cooking time: 10 minutes

Servings: 8

Ingredients:

- 16 ounces frozen broccoli florets, thawed
- 3 green onions, diced
- ½ teaspoon salt
- ¼ teaspoon ground black pepper
- 2 tablespoons soy sauce
- 1 tablespoon olive oil
- 1 ½ cups white rice, cooked

Directions:

1. Take a skillet pan, place it over medium heat, add broccoli, and cook for 5 minutes until tender-crisp.
2. Then add scallion and other ingredients, toss until well mixed and cook for 2 minutes until hot. Serve straight away.

Nutrition:

Calories: 187

Fat: 3.4 g

Carbs: 33 g

Protein: 6.3 g

106. Lentil, Rice and Vegetable Bake

Preparation time: 10 minutes

Cooking time: 40 minutes

Servings: 6

Ingredients:

- 1/2 cup white rice, cooked
- 1 cup red lentils, cooked
- 1/3 cup chopped carrots
- 1 medium tomato, chopped
- 1 small onion, peeled, chopped
- 1/3 cup chopped zucchini
- 1/3 cup chopped celery
- 1 ½ teaspoon minced garlic
- ½ teaspoon ground black pepper
- 1 teaspoon dried basil
- 1 teaspoon ground cumin
- 1 teaspoon dried oregano
- ½ teaspoon salt
- 1 teaspoon olive oil
- 8 ounces tomato sauce

Directions:

1. Take a skillet pan, place it over medium heat, add oil and when hot, add onion and garlic, and cook for 5 minutes.
2. Then add remaining vegetables, season with salt, black pepper, and half of each cumin, oregano and basil and cook for 5 minutes until vegetables are tender.
3. Take a casserole dish, place lentils and rice in it, top with vegetables, spread with tomato sauce and sprinkle with remaining cumin, oregano, and basil, and bake for 30 minutes until bubbly. Serve straight away.

Nutrition:

Calories: 187

Fat: 1.5 g

Carbs: 35.1 g

Protein: 9.7 g

107. Coconut Rice

Preparation time: 10 minutes

Cooking time: 25 minutes

Servings: 7

Ingredients:

- 2 ½ cups white rice
- 1/8 teaspoon salt
- 40 ounces coconut milk, unsweetened

Directions

1. Take a large saucepan, place it over medium heat, add all the ingredients in it and stir until mixed.
2. Boil the mixture, then switch heat to medium-low level and simmer rice for 25 minutes until tender and all the liquid is absorbed. Serve straight away.

Nutrition:

Calories: 535

Fat: 33.2 g

Carbs: 57 g

Protein: 8.1 g

108. Quinoa and Chickpeas Salad

Preparation time: 10 minutes

Cooking time: 0 minute

Servings: 4

Ingredients:

- 3/4 cup chopped broccoli
- 1/2 cup quinoa, cooked
- 15 ounces cooked chickpeas
- ½ teaspoon minced garlic
- 1/3 teaspoon ground black pepper
- 2/3 teaspoon salt
- 1 teaspoon dried tarragon
- 2 teaspoons mustard
- 1 tablespoon lemon juice
- 3 tablespoons olive oil

Directions:

1. Take a large bowl, place all the ingredients in it, and stir until well combined. Serve straight away.

Nutrition:

Calories: 264

Fat: 12.3 g

Carbs: 32 g

Protein: 7.1 g

109. Brown Rice Pilaf

Preparation time: 5 minutes

Cooking time: 25 minutes

Servings: 4

Ingredients:

- 1 cup cooked chickpeas
- 3/4 cup brown rice, cooked
- 1/4 cup chopped cashews
- 2 cups sliced mushrooms
- 2 carrots, sliced
- ½ teaspoon minced garlic

- 1 1/2 cups chopped white onion
- 3 tablespoons vegan butter
- ½ teaspoon salt
- ¼ teaspoon ground black pepper
- 1/4 cup chopped parsley

Directions:

1. Take a large skillet pan, place it over medium heat, add butter and when it melts, add onions and cook them for 5 minutes until softened.
2. Then add carrots and garlic, cook for 5 minutes, add mushrooms, cook for 10 minutes until browned, add chickpeas and cook for another minute.
3. When done, remove the pan from heat, add nuts, parsley, salt and black pepper, toss until mixed, and garnish with parsley. Serve straight away.

Nutrition:

Calories: 409

Fat: 17.1 g

Carbs: 54 g

Protein: 12.5 g

110. Barley and Mushrooms with Beans

Preparation time: 5 minutes

Cooking time: 15 minutes

Servings: 6

Ingredients:

- 1/2 cup uncooked barley
- 15 1/2 ounces white beans

- 1/2 cup chopped celery
- 3 cups sliced mushrooms
- 1 cup chopped white onion
- 1 teaspoon minced garlic
- 1 teaspoon olive oil
- 3 cups vegetable broth

Directions:

1. Put oil in your saucepan over medium heat, and when hot, add vegetables and cook for 5 minutes until tender.
2. Pour in broth, stir in barley, bring the mixture to boil, and then simmer for 50 minutes until tender.
3. When done, add beans into the barley mixture, stir until mixed and continue cooking for 5 minutes until hot. Serve straight away.

Nutrition:

Calories: 202

Fat: 2.1 g

Carbs: 39 g

Protein: 9.1 g

111. Vegan Curried Rice

Preparation time: 5 minutes

Cooking time: 25 minutes

Servings: 4

Ingredients:

- 1 cup white rice
- 1 tablespoon minced garlic
- 1 tablespoon ground curry powder
- 1/3 teaspoon ground black pepper

- 1 tablespoon red chili powder
- 1 tablespoon ground cumin
- 2 tablespoons olive oil
- 1 tablespoon soy sauce
- 1 cup vegetable broth

Directions:

1. Put oil in a saucepan over low heat, and when hot, add garlic and cook for 3 minutes.
2. Then stir in all spices, cook for 1 minute until fragrant, pour in the broth, and switch heat to a high level.
3. Stir in soy sauce, bring the mixture to boil, add rice, stir until mixed, then switch heat to the low level and simmer for 20 minutes until rice is tender and all the liquid has absorbed. Serve straight away.

Nutrition:

Calories: 262

Fat: 8 g

Carbs: 43 g

Protein: 5 g

112. Garlic and White Bean Soup

Preparation time: 15 minutes

Cooking time: 10 minutes

Servings: 4

Ingredients:

- 45 ounces cooked cannellini beans
- ¼ teaspoon dried thyme
- 2 teaspoons minced garlic

- 1/8 teaspoon crushed red pepper
- ½ teaspoon dried rosemary
- 1/8 teaspoon ground black pepper
- 2 tablespoons olive oil
- 4 cups vegetable broth

Directions:

1. Place one-third of white beans in a food processor, then pour in 2 cups broth and pulse for 2 minutes until smooth.
2. Place a pot over medium heat, add oil and when hot, add garlic and cook for 1 minute until fragrant.
3. Add pureed beans into the pan along with remaining beans, sprinkle with spices and herbs, pour in the broth, stir until combined, and bring the mixture to boil over medium-high heat.
4. Switch heat to medium-low level, simmer the beans for 15 minutes, and then mash them with a fork. Taste the soup to adjust seasoning and then serve.

Nutrition:

Calories: 222

Fat: 7 g

Carbs: 13 g

Protein: 11.2 g

113. Coconut Curry Lentils

Preparation time: 10 minutes

Cooking time: 40 minutes

Servings: 4

Ingredients:

- 1 cup brown lentils
- 1 small white onion, peeled, chopped
- 1 teaspoon minced garlic
- 1 teaspoon grated ginger
- 3 cups baby spinach
- 1 tablespoon curry powder
- 2 tablespoons olive oil
- 13 ounces coconut milk, unsweetened
- 2 cups vegetable broth

For Serving:

- 4 cups cooked rice
- ¼ cup chopped cilantro

Directions:

1. Put oil in your large pot over medium heat, and when hot, add ginger and garlic and cook for 1 minute until fragrant.
2. Add onion, cook for 5 minutes, stir in curry powder, cook for 1 minute until toasted, add lentils and pour in broth.
3. Switch heat to medium-high level, bring the mixture to a boil, then switch heat to the low level and simmer for 20 minutes until tender and all the liquid is absorbed.
4. Pour in milk, stir until combined, turn heat to medium level, and simmer for 10 minutes until thickened.
5. Remove the pot, stir in spinach, let it stand for 5 minutes until its leaves wilts and then top with cilantro. Serve lentils with rice.

Nutrition:

Calories: 184

Fat: 3.7 g

Carbs: 30 g

Protein: 11.3 g

114. Tomato, Kale, and White Bean Skillet

Preparation time: 10 minutes

Cooking time: 10 minutes

Servings: 4

Ingredients:

- 30 ounces cooked cannellini beans
- 3 1/2 ounces sun-dried tomatoes, chopped, packed in oil
- 6 ounces kale, chopped
- 1 teaspoon minced garlic
- 1/4 teaspoon ground black pepper
- 1/4 teaspoon salt
- 1/2 tablespoon dried basil
- 1/8 teaspoon red pepper flakes
- 1 tablespoon apple cider vinegar
- 1 tablespoon olive oil
- 2 tablespoons oil from sun-dried tomatoes

Directions:

1. Prepare the dressing and for this, place basil, black pepper, salt, vinegar, and red pepper flakes in a small bowl, add oil from sun-dried tomatoes and whisk until combined.
2. Take a skillet pan, place it over medium heat, add olive oil and when hot, add garlic and cook for 1 minute until fragrant.

3. Add kale, splash with some water and cook for 3 minutes until kale leaves have wilted. Add tomatoes and beans, stir well and cook for 3 minutes until heated.

4. Remove pan from heat, drizzle with the prepared dressing, toss until mixed and serve.

Nutrition:

Calories: 264

Fat: 12 g

Carbs: 38 g

Protein: 9 g

115. Chard Wraps with Millet

Preparation time: 25 minutes

Cooking time: 0 minute

Servings: 4

Ingredients:

- 1 carrot, cut into ribbons
- 1/2 cup millet, cooked
- 1/2 of a large cucumber, cut into ribbons
- 1/2 cup chickpeas, cooked
- 1 cup sliced cabbage
- 1/3 cup hummus
- Mint leaves as needed for topping
- Hemp seeds as needed for topping
- 1 bunch of Swiss rainbow chard

Directions:

1. Spread hummus on one side of chard, place some of millet, vegetables, and

chickpeas on it, sprinkle with some mint leaves and hemp seeds and wrap it like a burrito. Serve straight away.

Nutrition:

Calories: 152

Fat: 4.5 g

Carbs: 25 g

Protein: 3.5 g

116. Stuffed Peppers with Kidney Beans

Preparation time: 5 minutes

Cooking time: 35 minutes

Servings: 4

Ingredients:

- 3 1/2 ounces cooked kidney beans
- 1 big tomato, diced
- 3 1/2 ounces sweet corn, canned
- 2 medium bell peppers, deseeded, halved
- ½ of medium red onion, peeled, diced
- 1 teaspoon garlic powder
- 1/3 teaspoon ground black pepper
- 2/3 teaspoon salt
- ½ teaspoon dried basil
- 3 teaspoons parsley
- ½ teaspoon dried thyme
- 3 tablespoons cashew
- 1 teaspoon olive oil

Directions:

1. Switch on the oven, then set it to 400 degrees F and let it preheat. Take a large

skillet pan, place it over medium heat, add oil and when hot, add onion and cook for 2 minutes until translucent.

2. Add beans, tomatoes, and corn, stir in garlic and cashews and cook for 5 minutes.

3. Stir in salt, black pepper, parsley, basil, and thyme, remove the pan from heat and evenly divide the mixture between bell peppers. Bake the peppers for 25 minutes until tender, then top with parsley and serve.

Nutrition:

Calories: 139

Fat: 1.6 g

Carbs: 18 g

Protein: 5.1 g

117. Summer Harvest Pizza

Preparation Time: 20 minutes

Cooking Time: 15 minutes

Servings: 2

Ingredients:

- 1 lavash flatbread, whole grain
- 4 tbsp feta spread, store-bought
- ½ cup cheddar cheese, shredded
- ½ cup corn kernels, cooked
- ½ cup beans, cooked
- ½ cup fire-roasted red peppers, chopped

Directions:

1. Preheat oven to 350ºF. Cut Lavash into two halves. Bake crusts on a pan in the oven for 5 minutes.

2. Spread feta spread on both crusts. Top with remaining ingredients. Bake for another 10 minutes.

Nutrition:

Calories 230

Carbohydrates 23 g

Fats 15 g

Protein 11 g

118. Whole Wheat Pizza with Summer Produce

Preparation Time: 15 minutes

Cooking Time: 15 minutes

Servings: 2

Ingredients:

- 1 pound whole wheat pizza dough
- 4 ounces goat cheese
- 2/3 cup blueberries
- 2 ears corn, husked
- 2 yellow squash, sliced
- 2 tbsp olive oil

Directions:

1. Preheat the oven to 450°F. Roll the dough out to make a pizza crust.

2. Crumble the cheese on the crust. Spread remaining ingredients, then drizzle with olive oil. Bake for about 15 minutes. Serve.

Nutrition:

Calories 470

Carbohydrates 66 g

Fats 18 g

Protein 17 g

119. Tempeh Tikka Masala

Preparation time: 15 minutes

Cooking time: 20 minutes

Servings: 3

Ingredients:

Tempeh:

- ½ tsp sea salt

1 tsp of the following:

- garam masala
- ginger, ground
- cumin, ground
- 2 tsp apple cider vinegar
- ½ cup vegan yogurt
- 8 oz. tempeh, cubed

Tikka Masala Sauce:

- 2 cups frozen peas

1 cup of the following:

- full-fat coconut milk
- tomato sauce
- ¼ tsp turmeric
- ½ tsp sea salt
- 1 onion, chopped

1 tsp of the following:

- chili powder
- garam masala

- 1/4 cup ginger, freshly grated
- 3 cloves garlic, minced
- 1 tbsp. coconut oil

Directions:

1. Begin with making the tempeh by combining sea salt, garam masala, ginger, cumin, vinegar, and yogurt in a bowl. Add tempeh to the bowl and coat well; cover the bowl and refrigerate for 60 minutes.
2. In a pan big enough for 3 servings, add some coconut oil to heat using the medium setting, and begin preparing the sauce.
3. Sauté in the ginger, garlic, and onion for 5 minutes or until fragrant. Add the garam masala, chili powder, sea salt, and turmeric and combine well.
4. Add the frozen peas, coconut, milk, tomato sauce, and tempeh, reducing the heat to medium. Simmer within 15 minutes Remove from the heat and serve with cauliflower rice.

Nutrition:

Calories: 430

Carbohydrates: 39 g

Proteins: 21 g

Fats: 23 g

120. Caprice Casserole

Preparation time: 15 minutes

Cooking time: 37 minutes

Servings: 3

Ingredients:

Tempeh:

- ¼ cup basil, chopped
- 1 tomato, big
- ¼ tsp pepper
- ½ tsp salt

1 tbsp. of the following:

- nutritional yeast
- tahini
- 1 clove garlic
- 14 oz. tofu, extra firm, drained
- 6 cups marinara sauce
- 10 oz. vegetable noodles

Directions:

1. Set the oven to 350 heat setting. Cut the tofu into 4 slabs and remove excess moisture by gently squeezing each slab with a paper towel.
2. In a food processor, add garlic and chop, then scrape garlic from the sides to ensure it will be thoroughly mixed.
3. Add pepper, salt, yeast, tahini, and tofu to the food processor and pulse for 15 to 20 seconds until fully combined and forming a paste.
4. In an oven-safe dish, spread ½ cup of the marinara sauce across the bottom. Divide the vegetable noodles in half, break the noodles, and layer them on top of the sauce.
5. Put another layer of sauce over your noodles. Add the remaining noodles and coat the top with remaining sauce.

6. Using the tofu mixture from the food processor, form little patties about ½ thick and place on top of the sauce, filling up the dish.
7. Cover the baking container with aluminum foil and bake for 20 minutes. Uncover and bake again within 15 minutes.
8. Remove from the oven and set the oven to broil. Place the tomato slices on top of tofu mixture and broil for 2 minutes or until the tofu is lightly toasted. Garnish with basil. Serve warm and enjoy.

Nutrition:

Calories: 642

Carbohydrates: 88.6 g

Proteins: 25.1 g

Fats: 5.1 g

121. Cheesy Brussel Sprout Bake

Preparation time: 15 minutes

Cooking time: 46 minutes

Servings: 8

Ingredients:

- ½ onion sliced

2 tbsp. of each:

- garlic, chopped
- avocado oil
- 1 ½ lb. Brussel sprouts

Cheese:

- Dash cayenne

1 tsp of the following:

- onion powder
- salt

¼ tsp of the following:

- pepper
- paprika

½ tsp of the following:

- garlic, powder
- thyme
- 1 tbsp. tapioca starch
- ¼ cup nutritional yeast
- ½ cup vegetable broth
- 1 can coconut cream

Crumble Topping:

- ¼ tsp pepper
- ½ tsp garlic, powder
- 1 tsp salt
- ½ cup panko crumbs

Directions:

1. Bring the oven to 425 heat setting. Prepare Brussel sprouts by washing and trimming then steaming for 10 minutes.
2. Oiled an oven-safe baking dish with nonstick spray. Add the Brussel sprouts to a baking dish and set to the side.
3. Bring a skillet to medium temperature and mix in the garlic, avocado oil, and onion, sautéing approximately 6 minutes. Add the onion mixture to the top of the Brussel sprouts.
4. Put vegetable broth, nutritional yeast, onion powder, pepper, salt, garlic, paprika, thyme, and coconut cream in the same skillet on low heat, whisking together to combine.
5. Carefully add in the tapioca starch and whisk constantly; the mixture will thicken in about 5 minutes. Once it turns into a cheese sauce mixture, pour over the Brussel sprouts and onions.
6. In a mixing container, combine panko, salt, garlic, and pepper, creating the crumble. Sprinkle the crumble across the top of the cheese.
7. Cook in the oven within 25 minutes or until browned and golden. Serve warm and enjoy.

Nutrition:

Calories: 116

Carbohydrates: 16 g

Proteins: 4 g

Fats: 4 g

Chapter 8.   Dessert Recipes

122. Graham Pancakes

Preparation time: 15 minutes

Cooking time: 4 minutes

Servings: 6

Ingredients:

- 2 cups whole-wheat flour (about 11 ounces)
- 2 teaspoons baking powder
- ½ teaspoon baking soda
- 2 tablespoons date sugar
- ¾ teaspoon salt, optional
- 2½ cups unsweetened oat milk
- 2 tablespoons lemon juice
- ¼ cup unsweetened applesauce
- 2 teaspoons vanilla extract

Directions:

1. Combine the flour, baking powder and soda, date sugar, and salt (if desired) in a large bowl.
2. Make a well in the middle of the flour mixture, then add the oat milk, lemon juice, applesauce, and vanilla extract. Whisk the mixture until smooth and thick.
3. Make a pancake: Pour ¼ cup of the mixture in a nonstick skillet, then cook for 4 minutes. Flip the pancake halfway through the cooking time or until the first side is golden brown. Repeat with the remaining mixture. Transfer the pancakes on a plate and serve warm.

Nutrition:

Calories: 208

Fat: 3.1g

Carbs: 38.9g

Protein: 8.7g

123. Belgian Gold Waffles

Preparation time: 15 minutes

Cooking time: 5-6 minutes

Servings: 4

Ingredients:

- 2 cups soy flour (about 10 ounces)
- 1 tablespoon baking powder
- ¼ teaspoon baking soda
- 3 tablespoons cornstarch
- 2 tablespoons date sugar
- ½ teaspoon salt, optional
- 2 cups unsweetened soy milk
- 1 tablespoon lemon juice
- 1 teaspoon vanilla extract
- ¼ cup unsweetened applesauce

Directions:

1. Preheat the waffle iron. Combine the soy flour, baking powder and soda, cornstarch, date sugar, and salt (if desired) in a large bowl.
2. Make your well in the middle of the flour mixture, then add the soy milk, lemon juice, vanilla extract, and applesauce. Whisk the mixture until smooth and thick.
3. Add 1 cup of the mixture to the preheated waffle iron and cook for 5 to

6 minutes or until golden brown. Serve immediately. Repeat with the remaining mixture.

Nutrition:

Calories: 292

Fat: 8.0g

Carbs: 34.6g

Protein: 23.9g

124. Peach and Raspberry Crisp

Preparation time: 50 minutes

Cooking time: 30-35 minutes

Servings: 6

Ingredients:

Filling:

- 2½ pounds peaches, peeled, halved, pitted, and cut into ½-inch wedges
- ¼ cup maple sugar (about 1¾ ounces)
- 1/8 teaspoon salt, optional
- 1 tablespoon lemon juice
- 2 tablespoons ground tapioca
- 1 teaspoon vanilla extract
- 2 cups raspberries (about 10 ounces)

Topping:

- ½ cup soy flour (about 2½ ounces)
- ¼ teaspoon ground cinnamon
- ¼ teaspoon ground ginger
- ¼ cup date sugar (about 1¾ ounces)
- ¼ cup maple sugar (about 1¾ ounces)
- ¼ teaspoon salt, optional
- ¼ cup unsweetened applesauce
- ½ cup chopped pecans
- ½ cup rolled oats (about 1½ ounces)
- 2 tablespoons water

Directions:

Make the filling:

1. Warm your oven to 400ºF. Line a baking dish with parchment paper.
2. Put the peaches, maple sugar, and salt in a large bowl. Toss to combine well. Let stand for 30 minutes. Toss periodically.
3. Drain the peaches in a colander. Reserve 2 tablespoons of juice remain in the bowl and discard the extra juice.
4. Move the drained peaches back to the bowl. Add the lemon juice, tapioca, vanilla, and reserved peach juice. Toss to combine well.
5. Arrange the peaches and raspberries in the single layer on the baking dish.

Make the topping:

1. Put the soy flour, cinnamon, ginger, date sugar, maple sugar, and salt (if desired) in a food processor. Blitz for 15 seconds to combine well.
2. Add the applesauce to the mixture and blitz for 10 times until it becomes wet sand. Add the pecans, oats, and water and blitz for 15 times until smooth. Pour the batter in a large bowl then refrigerate for 20 minutes.
3. Spread the topping over the peaches and raspberries in the baking dish, then bake in the preheated oven for 30 to 35 minutes or until crispy and golden brown.

4. Flip the peaches and raspberries halfway through the cooking time. Remove the dish from the oven. Allow to cool within 30 minutes and serve.

Nutrition:

Calories: 294

Fat: 7.9g

Carbs: 55.9g

Protein: 7.7g

125. Chia Pudding with Coconut and Fruits

Preparation time: 15 minutes

Cooking time: 0 minutes

Servings: 4

Ingredients:

- 2 cups unsweetened soy milk
- 1½ teaspoons vanilla extract
- ½ cup chia seeds
- 2 tablespoons maple syrup
- ¼ teaspoon salt, optional
- ¼ cup flaked coconut, toasted
- 2 cups strawberries, avocado slices, and banana slices mix

Directions:

1. For the pudding, combine the soy milk, vanilla extract, chia seeds, maple syrup, and salt (if desired) in a bowl. Stir to mix well. Wrap your bowl in plastic then refrigerate for at least 8 hours.
2. Serve the pudding with coconut flakes and fruit mix on top.

Nutrition:

Calories: 303

Fat: 14.7g

Carbs: 36.0g

Protein: 9.5g

126. Orange and Cranberry Quinoa Bites

Preparation time: 25 minutes

Cooking time: 0 minutes

Servings: 12

Ingredients:

- 2 tablespoons almond butter
- 2 tablespoons maple syrup (optional)
- Zest of 1 orange
- 1 tablespoon dried cranberries
- ¾ cup cooked quinoa
- ¼ cup ground almonds
- 1 tablespoon chia seeds
- ¼ cup sesame seeds, toasted
- ½ teaspoon vanilla extract

Directions:

1. Mix the almond butter and maple syrup (if desired) in a medium bowl until smooth. Stir in the remaining ingredients, and mix to hold together in a ball.
2. Divide and form the mixture into 12 balls. Put them on a baking sheet lined with parchment paper. Put in the fridge to set for about 15 minutes. Serve chilled.

Nutrition:

Calories: 109

Fat: 11.0g

Carbs: 5.0g

Protein: 3.0g

127. Orange Glazed Bananas

Preparation time: 15 minutes

Cooking time: 4 minutes

Servings: 6-8

Ingredients:

- 1/3 cup fresh orange juice
- 6 ripe bananas, peeled and sliced
- 1 teaspoon vanilla extract
- ½ teaspoon ground cinnamon

Directions:

1. Put the orange juice in a saucepan and warm over medium heat. Add the sliced bananas and cook for 2 minutes.
2. Add the vanilla and cinnamon and continue to cook until the moisture is absorbed, about another 2 minutes. Serve warm.

Nutrition:

Calories: 98

Fat: 0.4g

Carbs: 24.7g

Protein: 1.2g

128. Pear Squares

Preparation time: 40 minutes

Cooking time: 50 minutes

Servings: 24 squares

Ingredients:

Filling:

- 1 (1-pound) can pears, with juice
- 2 cups chopped dried pears
- ¾ cup pitted dates
- ¼ cup tapioca
- 1 teaspoon orange extract

Crust:

- ½ cup pitted dates
- 1½ cups water
- ½ cup whole-wheat flour
- 1½ cups regular rolled oats
- 1/8 teaspoon salt (optional)
- 1 teaspoon vanilla extract

Topping:

- 1 cup regular rolled oats

Directions:

1. Put the canned pears and juice in a food processor and process until puréed. Transfer to a saucepan. Add the dried pears, dates, and tapioca. Simmer, covered, for 20 minutes. Add the orange extract and set aside.
2. Warm your oven to 375ºF. Combine the dates plus water in a food processor and process until finely ground.
3. In a bowl, combine the date water (reserve ¼ cup), flour, oats, salt (if desired), and vanilla. Press into a baking dish and bake for 10 minutes.

4. Meanwhile, toss the remaining rolled oats with the reserved date water. Spoon the filling over the crust. Sprinkle, the oat topping over the filling.

5. Bake in the preheated oven within 20 minutes, or until firm. Cool and cut into 2-inch squares before serving.

Nutrition:

Calories: 112

Fat: 0.8g

Carbs: 27.5g

Protein: 2.2g

129. Prune, Grapefruit, and Orange Compote

Preparation time: 15 minutes

Cooking time: 4 minutes

Servings: 4

Ingredients:

- 1 cup pitted prunes
- ¾ cup fresh orange juice
- 1 tablespoon maple syrup (optional)
- 2 (1-pound) cans unsweetened grapefruit sections, drained
- 2 (11-ounce) cans unsweetened mandarin oranges, drained

Directions:

1. Put the prunes, orange juice, and maple syrup (if desired) in a saucepan. Bring to a boil, reduce the heat, and cook gently for 1 minute. Remove from the heat and cool.

2. Combine the mixture with the grapefruit and mandarin oranges. Stir to mix. Cover and refrigerate for at least 2 hours before serving.

Nutrition:

Calories: 303

Fat: 0.7g

Carbs: 77.2g

Protein: 4.3g

130. Pumpkin Pie Squares

Preparation time: 15 minutes

Cooking time: 30 minutes

Servings: 16 squares

Ingredients:

- 1 cup unsweetened almond milk
- 1 teaspoon vanilla extract
- 7 ounces dates, pitted and chopped
- 1¼ cups old-fashioned rolled oats
- 2 teaspoons pumpkin pie spice
- 1 (15-ounce) can pure pumpkin

Directions:

1. Warm your oven to 375ºF (190ºC). Put the parchment paper in a baking pan. Stir together the milk and vanilla in a bowl. Soak the dates in it for 15 minutes, or until the dates become softened.

2. Add the rolled oats to a food processor and pulse the oats into flour. Remove the oat flour from the food processor

bowl and whisk together with the pumpkin pie spice in a different bowl.

3. Place the milk mixture into the food processor and process until smooth. Add the flour mixture and pumpkin to the food processor and pulse until the mixture has broken down into a chunky paste consistency.

4. Transfer the batter to the prepared pan and smooth the top with a silicone spatula. Bake within 30 minutes, or until a toothpick inserted in the center of the pie comes out clean. Let cool completely before cutting into squares. Serve cold.

Nutrition:

Calories: 68

Fat: 0.9g

Carbs: 16.8g

Protein: 2.3g

131. Apple Crisp

Preparation time: 15 minutes

Cooking time: 40 minutes

Servings: 6

Ingredients:

- ½ cup vegan butter
- 6 large apples, diced large
- 1 cup dried cranberries
- 2 tablespoons granulated sugar
- 2 teaspoons ground cinnamon, divided
- ¼ teaspoon ground nutmeg
- ¼ teaspoon ground ginger
- 2 teaspoons lemon juice
- 1 cup all-purpose flour
- 1 cup rolled oats
- 1 cup brown sugar
- ¼ teaspoon salt

Directions:

1. Preheat the oven to 350°F. Oiled an 8-inch square baking dish with butter or cooking spray.

2. Make the filling. In a large bowl, combine the apples, cranberries, granulated sugar, 1 teaspoon of cinnamon, the nutmeg, ginger, and lemon juice. Toss to coat. Transfer the apple mixture to the prepared baking dish.

3. Make the topping. In the same large bowl, now empty, combine the all-purpose flour, oats, brown sugar, and salt. Stir to combine.

4. Add the butter and, using a pastry cutter (or two knives moving in a crisscross pattern), cut the butter into the flour and oat mixture until the butter is the size of small peas.

5. Spread the topping over the apples evenly, patting down slightly. Bake for 40 minutes or until golden and bubbly.

Nutrition:

Calories: 488

Fat: 9 g

Carbs: 101 g

Protein: 5 g

132. Secret Ingredient Chocolate Brownies

Preparation time: 15 minutes

Cooking time: 35 minutes

Servings: 6-8

Ingredients:

- ¾ cup flour
- ¼ teaspoon baking soda
- ¼ teaspoon salt
- 1/3 cup vegan butter
- ¾ cup sugar
- 2 tablespoon water
- 1¼ cups semi-sweet or dark dairy-free chocolate chips
- 6 tablespoons aquafaba, divided
- 1 teaspoon vanilla extract

Directions:

1. Preheat the oven to 325°F. Line a 9-inch square baking pan with parchment or grease well. In a large bowl, combine the flour, baking soda, and salt. Set aside.
2. In a medium saucepan over medium-high heat, combine the butter, sugar, and water. Bring to a boil, stirring occasionally. Remove then stir in the chocolate chips.
3. Whisk in 3 tablespoons of aquafaba until thoroughly combined. Add the vanilla extract and the remaining 3 tablespoons of aquafaba, and whisk until mixed.
4. Add the chocolate mixture into the flour mixture and stir until combined. Pour in an even layer into the prepared pan.
5. Bake for 35 minutes, until the top is set but the brownie jiggles slightly when shaken. Allow to cool completely, 45 minutes to 1 hour, before removing and serving.

Nutrition:

Calories: 369

Fat: 19 g

Carbs: 48 g

Protein: 4 g

133. Chocolate Chip Pecan Cookies

Preparation time: 15 minutes

Cooking time: 16 minutes

Servings: 30 cookies

Ingredients:

- ¾ cup pecan halves, toasted
- 1 cup vegan butter
- ½ teaspoon salt
- ½ cup powdered sugar
- 2 teaspoons vanilla extract
- 2 cups all-purpose flour
- 1 cup mini dairy-free chocolate chips, such as Enjoy Life brand

Directions:

1. Preheat the oven to 350°F. Prepare a large rimmed baking sheet lined using parchment paper.

2. In a small skillet over medium heat, toast the pecans until warm and fragrant, about 2 minutes. Remove from the pan. Once these are cool, chop them into small pieces.

3. Combine the butter, salt, and powdered sugar, and cream using an electric hand mixer or a stand mixer fitted with a paddle attachment on high speed for 3 to 4 minutes, until light and fluffy. Add the vanilla extract and beat for 1 minute.

4. Turn the mixer on low and slowly add the flour, ½ cup at a time, until a dough form. Put the chocolate chips plus pecans, and mix until just incorporated.

5. Using your hands, a large spoon, or a 1-inch ice cream scoop, drop 1-inch balls of dough on the baking sheet, spaced 1 inch apart. Gently press down on the cookies to flatten them slightly.

6. Bake for 12 to 14 minutes until just golden around the edges. Cool on the baking sheet within 5 minutes before transferring them to a wire rack to cool. Serve or store in an airtight container.

Nutrition:

Calories: 152

Fat: 11 g

Carbs: 13 g

Protein: 2 g

134. Peanut Butter Chip Cookies

Preparation time: 15 minutes

Cooking time: 15 minutes

Servings: 12-15

Ingredients:

- 1 tablespoon ground flaxseed
- 3 tablespoons hot water
- 1 cup rolled oats
- 1 teaspoon baking soda
- 1 teaspoon ground cinnamon
- ¼ teaspoon salt
- 1 ripe banana, mashed
- ¼ cup maple syrup
- ½ cup all-natural smooth peanut butter
- 1 tablespoon vanilla extract
- ½ cup dairy-free chocolate chips

Directions:

1. Preheat the oven to 350°F. Prepare a large rimmed baking sheet lined using parchment paper.

2. Make a flaxseed egg by combining the ground flaxseed and hot water in a small bowl. Stir and let it sit for 5 minutes until thickened.

3. In a medium bowl, combine the oats, baking soda, cinnamon, and salt. Set aside.

4. Mash the banana then put the maple syrup, peanut butter, flaxseed egg, and vanilla extract in a large bowl. Stir to combine.

5. Add the dry batter into the wet batter and stir until just incorporated (do not overmix). Gently fold in the chocolate chips.

6. Using a large spoon or 2-inch ice cream scoop, drop the cookie dough balls onto the baking sheet. Flatten them slightly.

7. Bake within 12 to 15 minutes or until the bottoms and edges are slightly browned. Serve or store in an airtight container.

Nutrition:

Calories: 192

Fat: 12 g

Carbs: 17 g

Protein: 6 g

135. No-Bake Chocolate Coconut Energy Balls

Preparation time: 15 minutes

Cooking time: 0 minutes

Servings: 9

Ingredients:

- ¼ cup dry roasted or raw pumpkin seeds
- ¼ cup dry roasted or raw sunflower seeds
- ½ cup unsweetened shredded coconut
- 2 tablespoons chia seeds
- ¼ teaspoon salt
- 1½ tablespoons Dutch process cocoa powder
- ¼ cup rolled oats
- 2 tablespoons coconut oil, melted
- 6 pitted dates
- 2 tablespoons all-natural almond butter

Directions:

1. Combine the pumpkin seeds, sunflower seeds, coconut, chia seeds, salt, cocoa powder, and oats in a food processor or blender. Pulse until the mix is coarsely crumbled.
2. Add the coconut oil, dates, and almond butter. Pulse until the batter is combined and sticks when squeezed between your fingers.
3. Scoop out 2 tablespoons of mix at a time and roll them into 1½-inch balls with your hands. Place them spaced apart on a freezer-safe plate and freeze for 15 minutes.
4. Remove from the freezer and keep refrigerated in an airtight container for up to 4 days.

Nutrition:

Calories: 230

Fat: 12 g

Carbs: 27 g

Protein: 5 g

136. Blueberry Hand Pies

Preparation time: 15 minutes

Cooking time: 20 minutes

Servings: 6-8

Ingredients:

- 3 cups all-purpose flour, + extra for dusting work surface
- ½ teaspoon salt
- ¼ cup, plus 2 tablespoons granulated sugar, divided
- 1 cup vegan butter
- ½ cup cold water

- 1 cup fresh blueberries
- 2 teaspoons lemon zest
- 2 teaspoons lemon juice
- ¼ teaspoon ground cinnamon
- 1 teaspoon cornstarch
- ¼ cup unsweetened soy milk
- Coarse sugar, for sprinkling

Directions:

1. Warm your oven to 375°F. Prepare a large baking sheet lined using parchment paper. Set aside.
2. In a large bowl, combine the flour, salt, 2 tablespoons of granulated sugar, and vegan butter. Using a pastry cutter or two knives moving in a crisscross pattern, cut the butter into the other ingredients until the butter is the size of small peas.
3. Put the cold water then knead to form a dough. Tear the dough in half and wrap the halves separately in plastic wrap. Refrigerate for 15 minutes.
4. Make the blueberry filling. In a medium bowl, combine the blueberries, lemon zest, lemon juice, cinnamon, cornstarch, and the remaining ¼ cup of sugar.
5. Remove one half of the dough. On a floured surface, roll out the dough to ¼- to ½-inch thickness. Turn a 5-inch bowl upside down, and, using it as a guide, cut the dough into circles to make mini pie crusts.
6. Reroll scrap dough to cut out more circles. Repeat with the second half of the dough. You should end up with 10 to 12 circles. Place the circles on the prepared sheet pan.
7. Spoon 1½ tablespoons of blueberry filling onto each circle, leaving a ¼-inch border. Fold the circles in half to cover the filling, forming a half-moon shape. Press the edges of your dough to seal the pies using a fork.
8. When all the pies are assembled, use a paring knife to score the pies by cutting three lines through the top crusts.
9. Brush each pie with soy milk and sprinkle with coarse sugar. Bake for 20 minutes or until the filling is bubbly and the tops are golden. Let cool before serving.

Nutrition:

Calories: 416

Fat: 23 g

Carbs: 46 g

Protein: 6 g

137. Date Squares

Preparation time: 15 minutes

Cooking time: 25 minutes

Servings: 12

Ingredients:

- Cooking spray, for greasing
- 1½ cups rolled oats
- 1½ cups all-purpose flour
- ¾ cup, + 1/3 cup brown sugar, divided
- ½ teaspoon ground cinnamon
- ¼ teaspoon ground nutmeg

- 1 teaspoon baking soda
- ¼ teaspoon salt
- ¾ cup vegan butter
- 18 pitted dates
- 1 teaspoon lemon zest
- 1 teaspoon lemon juice
- 1 cup water

Directions:

1. Preheat the oven to 350°F. Oiled or spray a 9-inch square baking dish. Set aside.
2. Make the base and topping mixture. In a large bowl, combine the rolled oats, flour, ¾ cup of brown sugar, cinnamon, nutmeg, baking soda, and salt.
3. Add the butter and, using a pastry cutter or two knives working in a crisscross motion, cut the butter into the mixture to form a crumbly dough. Press half of your dough into the prepared baking dish and set the remaining half aside.
4. For the date filling, place a small saucepan over medium heat. Add the dates, the remaining 1/3 cup of sugar, the lemon zest, lemon juice, and water. Boil and cook within 7 to 10 minutes, until thickened.
5. When cooked, pour the date mixture over the dough base in the baking dish and top with the remaining crumb dough.
6. Gently press down and spread evenly to cover all the filling. Bake for 25 minutes until lightly golden on top. Cool before serving. Store in an airtight container.

Nutrition:

Calories: 443

Fat: 12 g

Carbs: 81 g

Protein: 5 g

138. Watermelon Lollies

Preparation Time: 15 minutes

Cooking Time: 0 minutes

Servings: 5

Ingredients:

- ½ cup watermelon, cubed
- 2 tablespoons lemon juice, freshly squeezed
- ½ cup water
- 1 tablespoon stevia

Directions:

1. In a food processor, put cubed watermelon. Process until smooth. Divide an equal amount of the mixture into an ice pop container. Place inside the freezer for 1 hour.
2. Meanwhile, in a small bowl, put together lemon juice, water, and stevia. Mix well. Pour over frozen watermelon lollies. Add in pop sticks. Freeze for another hour. Pry out watermelon lollies. Serve.

Nutrition:

Calories: 90

Carbs: 19g

Fat: 1g

Protein: 1g

139. Orange Blueberry Blast

Preparation Time: 30 minutes

Cooking Time: 0 minute

Servings: 1

Ingredients:

- 1 cup almond milk
- 1 scoop plant-based protein powder
- 1 cup blueberries
- 1 orange, peeled
- 1 teaspoon nutmeg
- 1 tablespoon shredded coconut

Directions:

1. Add all ingredients to a blender. Hit the pulse button and blend till it is smooth. Chill well to serve.

Nutrition

Calories: 155

Carbs: 12g

Fat: 21g

Protein: 1g

140. Chocolate Coconut Almond Tart

Preparation Time: 15 minutes

Cooking Time: 25 minutes

Servings: 9

Ingredients:

For crust:

- 1 cup almonds
- 2 tbsp. maple syrup
- 1 cup almond flour
- 3 tbsp. coconut oil

Filling & topping:

- 3 oz. bittersweet chocolate bars
- 1 tbsp. maple syrup
- oz. coconut milk
- Coconut, almonds
- Sea salt a pinch

Directions:

1. In a blender mix the almond flour and almonds until chopped and mix evenly. Pour maple syrup and coconut oil or mix well. Pour the batter into a baking pan and press it with a spoon to set its edges.
2. Bake the pie for 10 to 1 minutes in a preheated oven at 300 degrees until golden brown. Take a medium bowl, add chocolate and melt it over the boiling water. Add maple syrup on the top of the chocolate.
3. In a pan, add coconut milk and boil on a flame, pour the chocolate in boiling coconut milk and stir well until smooth.
4. Now pour the filling on the crust and top with almonds, coconut and sea salt. Store in a refrigerator for 2 hours or leave over the night. Serve the tart when completely set.

Nutrition:

Calories: 384

Carbs: 38g

Fat: 22g

Protein: 11g

141. Peanut Butter and Celery

Preparation Time: 5 minutes

Cooking Time: 0 minutes

Servings: 2

Ingredients:

- 4 stalks celery
- 1 cup peanut butter

Directions:

1. Take 4 stalks of celery, clean them well and let it dry. Now cut one stalk in 3 equal parts.
2. Apply the peanut butter with the knife on every stalk piece. Serve it with a cold glass of milk or enjoy a crunchy peanut butter celery.

Nutrition

Calories: 130

Carbs: 7g

Fat: 11g

Protein: 4g

Chapter 9.   Other Recipes

142. Avocado and Tempeh Bacon Wraps

Preparation time: 10 minutes

Cooking time: 8 minutes

Servings: 4

Ingredients:

- 2 tablespoons extra-virgin olive oil
- 8 ounces tempeh bacon, homemade or store-bought
- 4 (10-inch) soft flour tortillas or lavash flat bread
- ¼ cup vegan mayonnaise, homemade or store-bought
- 4 large lettuce leaves
- 2 ripe Hass avocados, pitted, peeled, and cut into ¼-inch slices
- 1 large ripe tomato, cut into ¼-inch slices

Directions:

- Heat-up the oil in a large skillet over medium heat. Add the tempeh bacon and cook until browned on both sides, about 8 minutes. Remove from the heat and set aside.
- Place 1 tortilla on a work surface. Spread with some of the mayonnaise and one-fourth of the lettuce and tomatoes.
- Thinly slice the avocado and place the slices on top of the tomato. Add the reserved tempeh bacon and roll up tightly. Repeat with remaining Ingredients and serve.

Nutrition:

Calories: 315

Carbs: 22g

Fat: 20g

Protein: 14g

143. Kale Chips

Preparation time: 5 minutes

Cooking time: 25 minutes

Servings: 2

Ingredients:

- 1 large bunch kale
- 1 tablespoon extra-virgin olive oil
- ½ teaspoon chipotle powder
- ½ teaspoon smoked paprika
- ¼ teaspoon salt

Directions:

- Preheat the oven to 275ºF. Prepare a large baking sheet lined using parchment paper. In a large bowl, stem the kale and tear it into bite-size pieces. Add the olive oil, chipotle powder, smoked paprika, and salt.
- Toss the kale with tongs or your hands, coating each piece well. Spread the kale over the parchment paper in a single layer.
- Bake within 25 minutes, turning halfway through, until crisp. Cool for 10 to 15 minutes before dividing and storing in 2 airtight containers.

Nutrition:

Calories: 100

Carbs: 9g

Fat: 7g

Protein: 4g

144. Tempeh-Pimiento Cheese Ball

Preparation time: 5 minutes

Cooking time: 30 minutes

Servings: 8

Ingredients:

- 8 ounces tempeh, cut into ½ -inch pieces
- 1 (2-ounce) jar chopped pimientos, drained
- ¼ cup nutritional yeast
- ¼ cup vegan mayonnaise, homemade or store-bought
- 2 tablespoons soy sauce
- ¾ cup chopped pecans

Directions:

Cook the tempeh within 30 minutes in a medium saucepan of simmering water. Set aside to cool. In a food processor, combine the cooled tempeh, pimientos, nutritional yeast, mayo, and soy sauce. Process until smooth.

Transfer the tempeh mixture to a bowl and refrigerate until firm and chilled for at least 2 hours or overnight.

Toast the pecans in a dry skillet over medium heat until lightly toasted. Set aside to cool.

Shape the tempeh batter into a ball, then roll it in the pecans, pressing the nuts slightly into the tempeh mixture so they

stick. Refrigerate within 1 hour before serving.

Nutrition:

Calories: 170

Carbs: 6g

Fat: 14g

Protein: 5g

145. Peppers and Hummus

Preparation time: 15 minutes

Cooking time: 0 minutes

Servings: 4

Ingredients:

- one 15-ounce can chickpeas, drained and rinsed
- juice of 1 lemon, or 1 tablespoon prepared lemon juice
- ¼ cup tahini
- 3 tablespoons extra-virgin olive oil
- ½ teaspoon ground cumin
- 1 tablespoon water
- ¼ teaspoon paprika
- 1 red bell pepper, sliced
- 1 green bell pepper, sliced
- 1 orange bell pepper, sliced

Directions:

Combine chickpeas, lemon juice, tahini, 2 tablespoons of the olive oil, the cumin, and water in a food processor.

Process on high speed until blended for about 30 seconds. Scoop the hummus into a bowl and drizzle with the remaining tablespoon of olive oil. Sprinkle with paprika and serve with sliced bell peppers.

Nutrition:

Calories: 170

Carbs: 13g

Fat: 12g

Protein: 4g

146. Roasted Chickpeas

Preparation time: 5 minutes

Cooking time: 25 minutes

Servings: 1 cup

Ingredients:

- 1 (14-ounce) can chickpeas, rinsed & drained/1½ cups cooked
- 2 tablespoons tamari, or soy sauce
- 1 tablespoon nutritional yeast
- 1 teaspoon smoked paprika, or regular paprika
- 1 teaspoon onion powder
- ½ teaspoon garlic powder

Directions:

Preheat the oven to 400°F. Toss the chickpeas with all the other fixings, and spread them out on a baking sheet.

Bake for 20-25 minutes, tossing halfway through. Bake these at a lower temperature until fully dried and crispy if you want to keep them longer.

You can easily double the batch, and if you dry them out they will keep about a week in an airtight container.

Nutrition:

Calories: 121

Fat: 2g

Carbs: 20g

Protein: 8g

147. Seed Crackers

Preparation time: 5 minutes

Cooking time: 50 minutes

Servings: 20

Ingredients:

- ¾ cup pumpkin seeds (pepitas)
- ½ cup sunflower seeds
- ½ cup sesame seeds
- ¼ cup chia seeds
- 1 teaspoon minced garlic (about 1 clove)
- 1 teaspoon tamari or soy sauce
- 1 teaspoon vegan Worcestershire sauce
- ½ teaspoon ground cayenne pepper
- ½ teaspoon dried oregano
- ½ cup water

Directions:

Preheat the oven to 325ºF. Prepare a rimmed baking sheet lined using parchment paper.

In a large bowl, combine the pumpkin seeds, sunflower seeds, sesame seeds, chia seeds, garlic, tamari,

Worcestershire sauce, cayenne,
oregano, and water.

Transfer to the prepared baking sheet and
spread it out to all sides. Bake for 25
minutes. Remove the pan, then flip the
seed "dough" over so the wet side is up.

Bake for another 20-25 minutes until the
sides are browned. Cool completely
before breaking up into 20 pieces.
Divide evenly among 4 glass jars and
close tightly with lids.

Nutrition:

Calories: 339

Fat: 29g

Protein: 14g

Carbohydrates: 17g

148. Tomato and Basil Bruschetta

Preparation time: 10 minutes

Cooking time: 6 minutes

Servings: 12

Ingredients:

3 tomatoes, chopped
¼ cup chopped fresh basil
1 tablespoon extra-virgin olive oil
pinch of sea salt
1 baguette, cut into 12 slices
1 garlic clove, sliced in half

Directions:

Combine the tomatoes, basil, olive oil, and
salt in a small bowl, and stir to mix. Set
aside. Preheat the oven to 425°F.

Put your baguette slices in a single layer on
your baking sheet and toast in the oven
until brown for about 6 minutes.

Flip the bread slices over once during
cooking. Remove from the oven and rub
the bread on both sides with the sliced
clove of garlic. Top with the tomato-
basil mixture and serve immediately.

Nutrition:

Calories: 102

Carbs: 17g

Fat: 3g

Protein: 0g

149. Refried Bean and Salsa Quesadillas

Preparation time: 5 minutes

Cooking time: 6 minutes

Servings: 4

Ingredients:

1 tablespoon canola oil, + more for frying
1½ cups cooked or 1 (15.5-ounce) can
pinto beans, drained and mashed
1 teaspoon chili powder
4 (10-inch) whole-wheat flour tortillas
1 cup tomato salsa, homemade or store-
bought
½ cup minced red onion (optional)

Directions:

In a medium saucepan, heat the oil over
medium heat. Add the mashed beans

and chili powder and cook, stirring, until hot, about 5 minutes. Set aside.

To assemble, place 1 tortilla on a work surface and spoon about ¼cup of the beans across the bottom half. Top the beans with the salsa and onion, if using. Fold top half of the tortilla over the filling and press slightly.

In large skillet heat a thin layer of oil over medium heat. Place folded quesadillas, 1 or 2 at a time, into the hot skillet and heat until hot, turning once, about 1 minute per side. Cut quesadillas into 3 or 4 wedges and arrange on plates. Serve immediately.

Nutrition:

Calories: 487

Carbs: 65g

Fat: 18g

Protein: 20g

150. Jicama and Guacamole

Preparation time: 15 minutes

Cooking time: 0 minutes

Servings: 4

Ingredients:

juice of 1 lime, or 1 tablespoon prepared lime juice

2 hass avocados, peeled, pits removed, and cut into cubes

½ teaspoon sea salt

½ red onion, minced

1 garlic clove, minced

¼ cup chopped cilantro (optional)

1 jicama bulb, peeled and cut into matchsticks

Directions:

In a medium bowl, squeeze the lime juice over the top of the avocado and sprinkle with salt. Lightly mash the avocado with a fork. Stir in the onion, garlic, and cilantro, if using.

Serve with slices of jicama to dip in guacamole. To store, place plastic wrap over the bowl of guacamole and refrigerate. The guacamole will keep for about 2 days.

Nutrition:

Calories: 145

Carbs: 0g

Fat: 10g

Protein: 9g

151. Tempeh Tantrum Burgers

Preparation time: 15 minutes

Cooking time: 14 minutes

Servings: 4

Ingredients:

8 ounces tempeh, cut into ½-inch dice

¾ cup chopped onion

2 garlic cloves, chopped

¾ cup chopped walnuts

½ cup old-fashioned or quick-cooking oats

1 tablespoon minced fresh parsley

½ teaspoon dried oregano

½ teaspoon dried thyme

½ teaspoon salt

¼ teaspoon freshly ground black pepper

3 tablespoons extra-virgin olive oil

Dijon mustard

4 whole grain burger rolls

Sliced red onion, tomato, lettuce, and
   avocado

Directions:

Cook the tempeh within 30 minutes in a
   medium saucepan of simmering water.
   Drain and set aside to cool.

Combine the onion and garlic in a food
   processor then process until minced.
   Put the cooled tempeh, the walnuts,
   oats, parsley, oregano, thyme, salt, and
   pepper. Process until well blended.
   Shape the mixture into 4 equal patties.

Heat-up the oil in a large skillet on medium
   heat. Add the burgers and cook until
   cooked thoroughly and browned on
   both sides for about 7 minutes per side.

Spread desired amount of mustard onto
   each half of the rolls and layer each roll
   with lettuce, tomato, red onion, and
   avocado as desired. Serve immediately.

Nutrition:

Calories: 150

Carbs: 8g

Fat: 7g

Protein: 13g

152. Sesame- Wonton Crisps

Preparation time: 15 minutes

Cooking time: 10 minutes

Servings: 12

Ingredients:

12 Vegan Wonton Wrappers

2 tablespoons toasted sesame oil

12 shiitake mushrooms, lightly rinsed,
   patted dry, stemmed, and cut into 1/4-
   inch slices

4 snow peas, trimmed and cut crosswise
   into thin slivers

1 teaspoon soy sauce

1 tablespoon fresh lime juice

½ teaspoon brown sugar

1 medium carrot, shredded

Toasted sesame seeds or black sesame
   seeds, if available

Directions:

Preheat the oven to 350°F. Oil a baking
   sheet and set aside. Brush the wonton
   wrappers with 1 tablespoon of the
   sesame oil and arrange on the baking
   sheet.

Bake until golden brown and crisp within 5
   minutes. Set aside to cool. (Alternately,
   you can tuck the wonton wrappers into
   mini-muffin tins to create cups for the
   filling. Brush with sesame oil and bake
   them until crisp.)

In a large skillet, heat the extra olive oil
   over medium heat. Add the mushrooms
   and cook until softened. Stir in the snow
   peas and the soy sauce and cook for 30
   seconds. Set aside to cool.

In a large bowl, combine the lime juice,
   sugar, and remaining 1 tablespoon

sesame oil. Stir in the carrot and cooled shiitake mixture.

Top each wonton crisp with a spoonful of the shiitake mixture. Sprinkle with sesame seeds and arrange on a platter to serve.

Nutrition:

Calories: 88

Carbs: 14g

Fat: 2g

Protein: 3g

153. Macadamia-Cashew Patties

Preparation time: 15 minutes

Cooking time: 10 minutes

Servings: 4

Ingredients:

¾ cup chopped macadamia nuts
¾ cup chopped cashews
1 medium carrot, grated
1 small onion, chopped
1 garlic clove, minced
1 jalapeño or other green chili, seeded and minced
¾ cup old-fashioned oats
¾ cup dry unseasoned bread crumbs
2 tablespoons minced fresh cilantro
½ teaspoon ground coriander
Salt and freshly ground black pepper
2 teaspoons fresh lime juice
Canola or grapeseed oil, for frying
4 sandwich rolls
Lettuce leaves and condiment of choice

Directions:

In a food processor, combine the macadamia nuts, cashews, carrot, onion, garlic, chili, oats, bread crumbs, cilantro, coriander, and salt and pepper.

Process until well mixed. Add the lime juice and process until well blended. Taste, adjusting the seasonings if necessary. Shape the mixture into 4 equal patties.

Heat-up a thin layer of oil in a large skillet over medium heat. Add the patties and cook until golden brown on both sides, turning once, for about 10 minutes in total. Serve on sandwich rolls with lettuce and condiments of choice.

Nutrition:

Calories: 190

Carbs: 7g

Fat: 17g

Protein: 4g

154. Lemon Coconut Cilantro Rolls

Preparation time: 60 minutes

Cooking time: 0 minutes

Servings: 16

Ingredients:

½ cup fresh cilantro, chopped
1 cup sprouts (clover, alfalfa)
1 garlic clove, pressed
2 tablespoons ground Brazil nuts or almonds
2 tablespoons flaked coconut
1 tablespoon coconut oil

Pinch cayenne pepper

Pinch sea salt

Pinch freshly ground black pepper

Zest and juice of 1 lemon

2 tablespoons ground flaxseed

1 to 2 tablespoons water

2 whole-wheat wraps, or corn wraps

Directions:

Put everything but the wraps in a food processor and pulse to combine. Or combine the fixings in a large bowl. Add the water, if needed, to help the mix come together.

Spread the mixture out over each wrap, roll it up, and place it in the fridge for 30 minutes to set.

Remove the rolls from the fridge and slice each into 8 pieces to serve as appetizers or sides with a soup or stew.

Get the best flavor by buying whole raw Brazil nuts or almonds, toasting them lightly in a dry skillet or toaster oven, then grinding them in a coffee grinder.

Nutrition:

Calories: 66

Fat: 4g

Carbs: 6g

Protein: 2g

155. Seeded Crackers

Preparation Time: 1 hour

Cooking Time: 10 minutes

Servings: 36 crackers

Ingredients:

½ cup pumpkin seeds
½ cup sunflower seeds
¼ cup sesame seeds
¼ cup chia seeds
¾ cup water
¾ teaspoon salt
1 teaspoon rosemary
1 teaspoon onion powder

Directions:

Preheat oven to 350°F. Set aside two large pieces of parchment paper. Combine all ingredients in a large bowl. Set aside to rest for 15 minutes.

Oil one side of each of the two sheets of parchment paper to avoid sticking in the next step.

Place the dough between the two pieces of parchment paper. Roll-out your dough thin using a rolling pin (roll to approximately 10 x 14 inch rectangle).

Slide the rolled out dough onto a baker's half sheet. Bake for 20 minutes. Remove from oven and cut into large pieces. Flip each piece over when finished. Bake for an additional 14 minutes. Serve.

Nutrition:

Calories 26

Fat 2 g

Protein 1 g

Carbs 2 g

Conclusion

Purple Plan has been used to help people lose weight and improve health. Michael Johnson, a bodybuilder who used the diet, claimed that he lost so much weight that he was able to shave off 30 pounds of fat and increase his lean muscle mass dramatically. According to Purple Plan reviews, the special plan does not have any negative side effects, and the only thing you feel is increased energy levels. It's also easier to follow than many other diets out there because you get to eat plenty of healthy apples.

Here is a FAQ to the Purple Plan:

1. What is Purple Plan?

Purple Plan is a dieting plan that combines the best features of two other dieting methods to produce the most effective and convenient way to lose weight: Intermittent Fasting and Ketosis. Along with these two powerful concepts, Purple Plan has one more important rule: No Red Foods!

2.What does Purple mean?

The 'Purple' part in this diet gives a hint about what you are supposed to eat. The Diet consists of 3 colors only. Purple, Green and White. Purple stands for Vegetables and meat, green stands for fruits, and white stands for dairy products.

3. What are the advantages of this diet plan?

Purple Plan is known to be incredibly easy to follow it is very similar to fasting, and keto style diets. The plan is designed in such a way that you can follow it as long as you wish. It is thought that the best results can be obtained when the diet is followed for no longer than 1 month at a time. This diet plan is easy to follow and very satisfying.

4. How does Purple Plan work?

The body of a person who adapts to Purple Plan works in an incredibly efficient way. In brief:

Intermittent Fasting- The method of intermittent fasting helps stimulate your body and allow it to reach a state of ketosis which leads to weight loss. Ketosis is a state when your body produces more ketones than it needs to use as energy. Ketones are created in the liver after fats are broken down during fasting.

5. What do I eat on Purple Plan?

There is only one thing you have to consume on this diet: healthy fruits, vegetables, meat and dairy products (not including foods with high level of sugar content).

6. What is the difference between Purple Plan and other dieting plans?

The most important difference is that Purple Plan focuses on healthy food instead of the number of calories you consume. You can eat all the nutritious food that your body desires. The difference in this diet plan is that you don't need to count calories or portion sizes, which allows you to better monitor how much and what types of food you are eating.

7. Where Can I buy Purple Plan?

The best place to buy this diet plan is from their official website.

8. Why is Purple Plan the best diet plan for me?

Purple Plan is a diet plan that has been around for years and has proven to be effective in many people. The unique combination of intermittent fasting and ketosis makes this diet completely different from others out there. Many people have tried other diets and failed, not because they didn't work but because they were hard to follow or complicated for some reason.

The Purple Plan is a weight loss diet that can help you achieve any weight management goals. The system is based on a unique family of 12 food categories, which are all color-coded. This blog post will discuss how to use the program by illustrating how to order breakfast through lunch for one day using the various Purple Plan food categories.

In conclusion, purple plan is a diet that aids in maintaining good health and weight loss. People who go on this diet will experience many positive changes in their bodies as well as their overall wellbeing.

Printed in Great Britain
by Amazon